DIETING:

A DRY DRUNK

by

Becky Lu Jackson

Universal Publishers

Universal Publishers / uPUBLISH.com

USA • 2000

ISBN: 1-58112-708-1

www.upublish.com/books/jacksonb.htm

Printing History

BLJ Nautilus Publications / 11/91

DEDICATION

This book is dedicated to

my daughter Laura
my son Jeff
It was through my love for them
that I began my recovery

all the compulsive overeaters
who have shared the path of
recovery with me

all the compulsive overeaters
still suffering—join us now

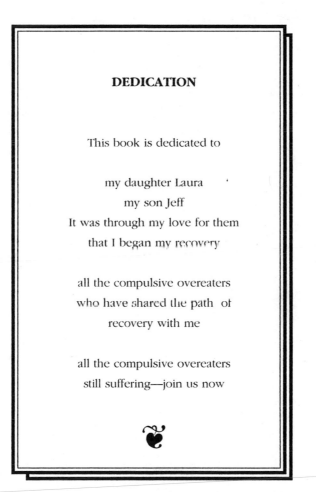

ACKNOWLEDGEMENTS

A special thanks to John Haehl for encouraging me to dream and believing in me; Miriam Harris for being my first "Grandma;" Judy Bluestone for teaching me to talk from my heart; Sharon James for laughter and love; Ronald Ballegeer for all his conscious and unconscious pushes toward growth; and a special acknowledgement to my children, Laura Ballegeer and Jeff Ballegeer, who have given me an opportunity to practice living by spiritual principles and to experience unconditional love, they have been the joy and the love of my life. Finally, I want to thank my Higher Power for the interesting, challenging and joyous path I've been privileged to walk this lifetime.

FOREWORD

Eating disorders are biological illnesses like diabetes and heart disease. Compulsive eating, anorexia, and bulimia do **not** occur because of lack of will power or personality flaws. Research is finding that people with eating disorders have chemical differences within the brain that make it likely that they will eat abnormally. Just as we cannot cure diabetes or heart disease, we cannot cure an eating disorder. Just as someone with heart disease must take special care of themselves *because* of their disease, so must a person with an eating disorder. Otherwise, the disease gets worse and, tragically, often kills. This book is a desperately needed step-by-step guide to how a person with an eating disorder can take care of themselves.

Every person with an eating disorder has asked "Why me?" There are surely those who have the chemical imbalances that put them at risk for an eating disorder, but never develop one. Eating disorders occur when the chemical imbalance is brought out by confusion, stress, and most of all, painful feelings. For everyone with an eating disorder, the cycle started with pain. Full recovery means walking through the pain and letting go of the shame and old beliefs about not being good enough.

Unfortunately, no one can functionally deal with pain when their lives are unmanageable and when the eating disorder is out of control. This book is about getting control of an unmanageable life. As a psychiatrist, I have learned a great deal from Becky Jackson about how to treat patients with eating disorders. I have applied her insights to my own patients and have realized results that did not occur before. Now all of my patients follow her guidelines to arrest the disorder *first* and *then* we work on the painful feelings underneath.

None of us as psychiatrists or counselors can fix a person with an eating disorder. While there is hope that better medicines will be developed (some already help) and we will learn how to serve as better guides to recovery, people with eating disorders must fix themselves. They must admit that they are sick, that their lives are out of control and start *living* the tools to recovery.

This book comes from the years of experience and hard work of a woman who has systematically taken the steps to recover from an illness that almost took her life. Now, in full recovery, she has been a guide and teacher to many whose lives were destroyed by their inability to eat sanely and moderately. The methods that worked for her, worked for them, too. Because her system works, this book will be a source of inspiration to the millions of women and men who live in the despair and shame of eating disorders.

I want to recommend this book as required reading for those with eating disorders, their families, friends and therapists. It is not based on speculation. It is based on facts and success. The message of this book is that there is no easy way to recovery, but *there is a way to recover*. Reading this will not make anyone well. **Living** the book and **living** the recovery, will.

Becky has learned to love herself and get well in the process. Loving oneself is tougher than it seems. But recovery starts there. This book is her story but the recovery can apply to all who live it.

Joseph Mortola, M.D.

INTRODUCTION

This book is for people with eating problems and weight problems. It's for those who have experienced obsessive and compulsive attempts to control their weight and their eating. It's for people who have failed at achieving weight control and eating stability through fad diets, behavior modification methods, nutritional guidance and insight oriented therapy.

It's not wishy-washy; it's not esoteric. It introduces a solution that is simple yet radically new to the chronic dieting/weight controlling subculture. It outlines, at present, scientifically unproven ideas and concepts. Even though there is research being done at this time that might confirm and support the concepts I present here, the facts are that I have personally experienced the benefits of using them in my own life since '74 and over the years I have observed the benefits others have experienced when applying them to their own lives.

I present and explain the concept of eating disorders as an addictive disease. Applying the addictive disease concept to eating disorders offers clarity about the recovery process. Using this philosophy creates hope for permanent recovery from all expressions of eating disorders—obesity, starving, grazing, purging, and restricting.

This is a book about *how's*—not whys—*how* to arrest an eating disorder a day at a time, *how* to stop the damaging dynamics, *how* to live free of the compulsions and obsessions, *how* to identify and let go of the dieting mentality, *how* we've used our eating, our weight/shape and our obsessional thinking to deal with life, and *how* to live free of the need for our illness.

It doesn't focus on the "what am I eating over" or "why I ate" questions. It explains through an analogy with alcoholism, that when an addictive disease is present, pursuing the "whys" erroneously implies that if a good enough explanation is presented *then* the destructive actions are acceptable and/or justifiable.

Attempting to use willpower and self-awareness to bring an addictive disease under control results in repeated failures. For people with eating disorders, these repeated failures push us toward adopting controlling methods that are physically and mentally damaging, methods such as compulsive exercising, starving with and without diet pills, vomiting, laxative and/or diuretic abuse, and sometimes even cosmetic surgery.

The solution concepts speak to a **recovery mentality**; accepting the need for a "bottom line," accessing a new relationship with honesty and moderation, identifying reality about body image and maintenance weight, preparing for the prevention of relapse, and understanding how we've used our eating and weight issues for protection and manipulation. They are outlined in a handbook style with definitions and exercises.

The "12-Step answer" that is available in Alcoholics Anonymous and Overeaters Anonymous literature and meetings is suggested as ongoing, follow-up support.

These new perceptions and new solutions are presented through short, easy to read chapters. The short, simple chapters are sprinkled with personal anecdotes and include personal recovery stories, my own as the first story of Part II. The personal recovery stories emphasize and reflect the benefits of applying these basic concepts.

My goals for the book are:

- to explain why relief from the exhausting and consuming cycle of on and off weight and food controlling has eluded so many

- to present a recovery path

- to bring hope and clarity about possibility of permanent recovery for the suffering problem eater.

I believe this book can make a difference. It could be the last dieting book that the millions of chronic dieters buy as a "fix it" book. The beliefs, concepts, attitudes and behaviors outlined, if sincerely embraced, can create positive change and guide the problem eater to the status of living a happy and usefully whole life—a life free from a compulsive, obsessive relationship with food, eating and body image.

DIETING: A DRY DRUNK

CONTENTS

PART I

UNDERSTANDING EATING DISORDERS. 1

   a. keys to identify: control, obsession, denial

   b. addictive disease description

   c. eating disorder description

WHY "NO RANDOM EATING"? 10

   a. dieting feeds obsession

   b. giving up the option - giving up the obsession

   c. definition of "random eating"

DIETING MENTALITY 13

   a. subtle attitudes

   b. subtle behavior

   c. subtle danger

WHAT'S BLACK & WHITE & WHAT'S GREY 16

   a. finding a bottom line equal to sobriety

   b. making the black & white achievable 100% of the time

   c. finding flexibility (the grey) & when & how it's useful

THE DANGER OF LIVING IN THE GREY 19

   a. examples of "grey" behavior

   b. consequences of abusing flexibility of abstinence

RECEIVING THE OA MESSAGE 21

   a. epilepsy analogy

   b. treatment centers and AA's 12 Steps

   c. locating OA near you

MODERATE IS MODERATE IS MODERATE 25

    a. moderate is a recovery issue

    b. moderate is a health issue

    c. moderate is a relapse issue

ONE MEAL AT A TIME, ONE DAY AT A TIME 29

    a. the 24-hour plan

    b. the 1-hour plan

    c. the 1-minute plan

DOES IT FEED THE DISEASE OR DOES IT FEED THE RECOVERY? 32

    a. the set-up of relapse energy

    b. how to decide on actions that bring serenity

    c. examples of disease calming actions

KEEPING IT SIMPLE 34

    a. analysis paralysis

    b. do what's in front of you

    c. using slogans

WATCH OUT FOR THE "PINK CLOUD" 36

    a. overelation often a danger signal

    b. "never have it made" concept

THE GREAT OBSESSION 38

    a. alcoholism analogy

    b. hidden belief about therapy

    c. acceptance

SEEKING PROFESSIONAL HELP 40

    a. types to assist recovery

    b. no perfect people/us or them

    c. ultimately our responsibility

INSTITUTIONAL MENTALITY 42

    a. subtle attitudes

    b. subtle behavior

    c. subtle danger

WHAT ABOUT EXERCISE? 45

    a. much needed in moderation

    b. suggestions for either extreme

    c. potential dangers of body sculpturing

EAT TO NOURISH, NOT CONTROL 48

    a. give up dieting & control

    b. American Heart Assoc. guidelines

    c. definition of healthy eating achievable 75% of the time

    d. 4 nutritional tips

MAINTENANCE: WHAT A CONCEPT 52

    a. abstaining vs dieting

    b. key recovery issue

    c. pitfalls to watch for

    d. suggestions

SURRENDER TO WIN . . . PARDON ME? 59

    A. outside changes don't take "it" away

    b. "hitting bottom" = giving up the losing fight

    c. stopping the war = winning

CHANGING OLD ROUTINES. 61

    a. old behavior leads to old results

    b. new behavior leads to new results

    c. types of things to change in the beginning

FIRST THINGS FIRST 64

   a. recovery a matter of survival

   b. keep perspective, not perfection

   c. must cherish self to cherish others

H.A.L.T. (Hungry, Angry, Lonely, Tired) 66

   a. define acronym

   b. pitfall of each

   c. need for balance

BEING PREPARED FOR SOCIAL OCCASIONS 69

   a. plan, alternate plan, let go of results

   b. decide in advance stops obsession

   c. add to life stops self obsession

KNOW YOUR RELAPSE INDICATORS 73

   a. emotional relapse precedes physical

   b. examples of common ones

   c. know yours and make a plan

   d. prevention work with body image issues

BODY IMAGE: #1 RELAPSE PROBLEM 80

   a. used to set "boundaries"

   b. "looks are for looking at" concept

   c. self-hate manifests in the mirror

   d. must resolve for recovery

INNER FAMILY HEALING 85

   a. "How we've used our disease" concept

   b. "inner family" description

   c. visualization suggestion

   d. codependency enmeshment

FIND, DEVELOP, AND USE A SUPPORT SYSTEM 89
    a. list of ideas to help develop support system
    b. understanding why immediate family might not
       be best choice for support

LOOKING FOR "GRANDMAS" 91
    a. definition of a "Grandma"
    b. importance of one
    c. what to look for

REMEMBER YOUR LAST DIET &/OR BINGE 93
    a. selective recall problem
    b. remembering the before, during and after
    c. use memories to aid change

EMOTIONS DON'T DEMAND ACTIONS 95
    a. emotions are not random, connected to beliefs
    b. change perceptions, change feelings
    c. "neither yield nor resist"

READING YOUR RICHTER SCALE 98
    a. overreaction means old reaction
    b. humorous examples
    c. key to old idea - key to new idea

IS THERE LIFE AFTER ABSTINENCE 101
    a. loss of an old "friend"
    b. fear of success: letting go of excuses
    c. facing the shame of "why haven't you ...."
    d. healing the past to move forward
    e. free to go for our dreams

PART II

10 PERSONAL SUCCESS STORIES

FROM THE AUTHOR 107
    a. my history
    b. my recovery & my pain
    c. my insights & my hope for others

MARGO C. — YOU CAN'T GET THERE FROM HERE 120

JEANIE M. — NEVER LOSE HOPE 130

LISA M. — BEAUTY AND BRAINS COULDN'T HELP 141

STEVEN M. — THE WAY OUT 151

TERI K. — FULL RECOVERY, FULL LIFE 160

JEAN M. — FROM DIETING MADNESS TO DISEASE RECOVERY 169

JERRY J. — RECOVERY FROM SELF-WILL RUN RIOT 175

KATHY R. — I THOUGHT I HAD TO BE OLD 183

LAURA B. — I WASN'T READY 189

PART I

CHAPTER 1
UNDERSTANDING EATING DISORDERS

Understanding that an addictive disease has been the driving energy behind our eating/weight problems can bring a sense of astonishment. Additionally, understanding the dynamics of that disease can bring us an accepting, calm view of ourselves for the first time in years. That acceptance and understanding can result in relief, *if* we also hear there is a way to arrest it—a way to recover.

The information available about alcoholism as an addictive disease and the possibility of recovery—not just *"getting better"*—led the way for my concepts about eating disorders and eating disorder recovery. In sharing that new perspective with you, a different view of the struggle with dieting and weight control will unfold, I will explain the concept of eating disorders as an addictive disease. Concrete tools will be presented to assist your path of recovery. I will introduce you to the concept of an *"inner family."* Your younger, historical selves who have an attachment to the eating disorder will be invited to let go of the belief that they **need the disease.**

Behind the concept that eating disorders are an illness, not a will power issue, are three basic beliefs; **one**, that *you have a disease, but you're not the disease,* **two**, that *the eating disorder is not simply a dysfunctional coping mechanism,* and **three**, *awareness and knowledge about your eating disorder implies responsibility for recovery from the disease.* In presenting these central concepts, I hope to create a framework filled with tools, ideas, suggestions and beliefs that will offer you relief from the damaging cycle of dieting, controlling and failure—that offer you stable, permanent recovery from the eating disorder.

Many of the concepts, insights and ideas came directly from my personal attempts to apply my understanding about alcoholism to my own eating problem. Many came from Overeaters Anonymous literature (an organization similar to Alcoholics Anonymous). Many came from watching and helping others discover their own answers while we all trudged down recovery's road.

I believe that eating disorders can be arrested, although not cured, and that there is hope for stable recovery and permanent change. I want to help you design a "*recovery mentality*" with which to approach food, weight, eating issues—with which to approach life.

Addictive Disease/Eating Disorder Characteristics

In clarifying the position that eating disorders are in the addictive disease category, I use alcoholism as an analogy because it's the most commonly understood addictive disease.

Alcoholism is characterized by:

- Compulsion
- Loss of Control
- "Repeated Use" (attempts to control) In Spite of Adverse Consequences

Eating Disorders are characterized by:

- **Compulsion/obsession**—an irrational driving need to eat and/or an irrational driving need to control body weight and shape manifested in a persistent, disturbing preoccupation with eating/food/weight/body image.

- Progressive **loss of control**—chronic obesity, chronic dieting, addictive purging and/or starving

- **Repeated use** (or *attempts to control*) in spite of adverse consequences—attempts to control eating, body weight and shape through dieting, attempts to over-control through restricting, severe restricting and starving, with or without diet pill use/abuse and attempts to eliminate the consequences of out-of-control eating through various forms of purging (vomiting, excessive exercising, laxative abuse, diuretic abuse and/or a combination of these), without regard or even recognition of the consequences of such actions on our minds and bodies. These repeated attempts, without regard for the physical, emotional and spiritual consequences reflect a large dose of **denial**.

Addictive Disease/Eating Disorder Mind-Sets

There are also three major mind-sets to addictive diseases, **denial, obsession, and control.** These mental postures map absolutely on the major characteristics of eating disorders.

Denial is the first mental characteristic of an eating disorder. If you have this illness, the first thing you will tell yourself is that you *don't* have this illness. You only have a temporary problem. Just as soon as you get to your ideal weight or get rid of the stress in your life **then** it will be easy to eat the "*right*" way, **then** it will no longer be a problem. Or you tell yourself, you didn't grow up with a weight problem, so the "right" nutritional guidance will solve this temporary situation.

We desperately want to be like others—not *weak willed* or immature. Because our society typically views obesity and out-of-control eating as a moral, or worse yet, an emotional weakness, we feel driven to deny the fact that we belong in this category. In our struggle to deny having this baffling "*defect*," we deny having the disease. When we deny having the eating disorder, by default, we eliminate the possibility of recovery. We stay hopelessly caught in the struggle.

But if we get rigorously honest, we can usually admit that we ate when we were stressed *and* when we were bored, we ate when sad and lonely *as well as* during happy celebrating. We ate compulsively in the best of times and the worst of times and sometimes for no rational, understandable reason at all. This describes an **addiction**, feeling driven to do it *even* when every ounce of rational thought doesn't want to. Addictive diseases are cunning, baffling and powerful.

The second mental posture is *obsession*—obsession with eating, with food, with body image, with nutrition, with health, with exercise, *and* obsession with **control**. The dictionary describes obsession as a persistent, preoccupation with an idea and/or a feeling. Although, we have probably benefited in the past from using our obsessional thinking to avoid painful situations and feelings, in reality our obsessions have interfered with our productivity, our creativity, our sanity and our relationships with others. It has interfered with our ability to live a peaceful life.

Unlike alcoholism which typically has only one primary obsession, the obsession to drink, eating disorders generally manifest themselves in three primary obsessions:

- the obsession with eating
- the obsession with food
- the obsession with body weight and shape

Although the primary obsessions might feel equal in their devastation, the eating compulsion/obsession will need to be addressed first. It will need to be addressed and arrested first because the *compulsion*—the acting out behavior—has to be stopped to clearly and sanely address the remaining obsessions and accompanying recovery issues.

The third major mind-set is **control**—planning and wanting to control our weight and our eating. The periods when we experience *loss of control* increases our wanting and planning to get *control*. Recall trying to gain control of your eating/weight problem through dieting, dieting institutions/centers, nutritional guidance, health spas, starving, purging and trips to doctors and therapists, only to inevitably re-experience loss of control. Our failures are eventually followed by more wanting and planning to acquire "permanent" control. These attempts to control often result in our weight "*yo-yo'ing*" up and down, and eventually, over time, it can result in the feeling of total loss of control, meaning we no longer feel we have the ability or energy to try the newest weight control plan.

As time (and the disease) progresses, even our mini-attempts to just get from lunch to dinner fail. We often feel such despair that we settle for only wanting control—we've given up the planning. Interestingly, the hopelessness and despair can become our greatest ally. It can be a "*bottom*" that sets the stage for a new kind of honesty, open-mindedness and willingness—for recovery.

Arresting an Addictive Disease/Eating Disorder

To arrest an addictive disease—*our eating disorder*—we will need a "bottom line." For an alcoholic, that bottom line is no drinking alcohol. It's called **sobriety**. For a drug addict, that bottom line is no use of mind-altering drugs. It's called **clean**. Eating disorder sufferers desperately need that rock solid, clear as a bell, foundation of a bottom line too. That primary compulsion/obsession to overeat and/or restrict our food over anything, everything and/or nothing, **must not be acted on**. It's called **abstinence**, meaning abstaining from compulsive, impulsive, random eating in between meals and no overeating/undereating at the meals.

The book <u>Overeaters Anonymous</u> says, "We practice abstinence by staying away from all eating between planned meals. . ." O.A. labels the disease "compulsive overeating." Implying that the illness has two major components, *compulsiveness* and *overeating* (volume consumption).

I tend to agree with the O.A. philosophy, the core of the illness is compulsive overeating. We may attempt to control the overeating through dieting/restricting or attempt to eliminate the consequences of overeating through some form of purging **but** the core is compulsive overeating. Both the compulsiveness and the overeating need to be addressed in our definition of abstinence. Through O.A.'s use of the word "planned," they attempt to address the dangerous compulsive, impulsive energy. And the word "meal" implies a moderate serving of food—not a junior banquet and not a starvation/diet serving.

In the first few months of my own abstinence, the behavioral expression of meal planning was pretty detailed. When I planned what the meals were going to be for the 24 hour period in front of me, the obsessions seemed to be quieted. But further in to my abstinence, the planning took a less detailed expression—I plan on eating breakfast, I plan on eating lunch and I plan on eating dinner, I plan on eating moderate. And on rare occasions, I have a day where the plan is to eat brunch and dinner. Although, without exception, both the meals are always in the moderate range.

Finally understanding that "*random*" **is** the factor that triggers the compulsive eating frenzy brings clarity to our bottom line. When we **give up the option** to randomly eat in between moderate meals, *or* randomly add on extra food at our meals, *or* randomly skip meals, the driving compulsive energy miraculously begins to vanish. The thoughts to eat in between meals or to start randomly reducing or adding on extra food to a moderate meal might drift through our mind from time to time but they no longer carry the obsessive quality. We're no longer taking them seriously when we're committed to our bottom line of avoiding compulsive, impulsive, random eating.

The obsessive mind-set is about options—the "will I or won't I, should I or shouldn't I" dilemma. The obsessive thinking will begin to dissipate once we let go of the option of **whether or not** to take our "medicine" of abstinence. Once we are committed to *no random eating in between moderate meals, no matter what*, we begin to experience some freedom—freedom from the compulsion and obsession.

Just as the alcoholic experiences a clarity of mind and emotions from continuous sobriety, we experience the clarity of mind and emotions that comes from continuous abstinence, thus making it finally possible to address the other primary obsessions, as well as the other related recovery issues.

The *food obsession* and the *body image obsession* are multifaceted and are best taken piecemeal, one insight, one awareness, one change at a time *(and in this book, one chapter at a time)*. But in recovery, arresting the compulsions **first** is crucial.

The three **secondary** obsessions typically connected with eating disorders are:

- the obsession with nutrition
- the obsession with health
- the obsession with exercise

These usually got set into motion through our "attempts to control"—attempts to control the driving need to eat and/or the attempts to control the consequences of out-of-control eating.

Purging—deliberate elimination of calories or food—usually starts out as an attempt to avoid the consequences of overeating or bingeing. It can also become a compulsion/obsession, sometimes of primary status, sometimes secondary. Often times we use it as an attempt to control body shape and size; sometimes we live the delusion that it can relieve stress. Again, purging can include vomiting, excessive exercising, laxative abuse, diuretic abuse, and/or a combination of these. Intentionally getting rid of calories is a simple definition of purging. If purging has also become an addiction—a **"process addiction"**—we'll need to **get and keep a bottom line for it too**.

These descriptions put an umbrella over all expressions of eating disorders—chronic yo-yo dieting, chronic restricting/starving, chronic obesity, chronic purging and/or any mix of the different expressions. All expressions typically stem from the compulsion—the driving, irrational need to eat.

In 1974 I began interacting with and observing people with eating disorders. It appears apparent to me that most expressions of eating disorders consist of a combination of ingredients, a **biological predisposition** to develop the eating disorder, **unconsciously perceived benefits** of the disease and **process addictions**.

To date, there is some very good information available about process addictions. Compulsive gambling, compulsive spending and compulsive shopping would be categorized as process addictions; they do not involve ingesting or injecting a substance into the body. The pay off (or high) comes from the **process of performing a series of ritualized behaviors.**

Substance addictions, such as cocaine and heroin, typically have a large component of process addiction in them. The physiological changes that take place during the ritualistic behaviors that *precede* ingestion or injection of the drug creates a similar "*rush*" **prior** to the drug induced rush. For the alcoholic, the process addiction rush might be triggered by entering a liquor store to purchase a bottle or by simply getting dressed for a night out on the town.

Dieting, bingeing, grazing and purging all have the possibility of ritualized actions—they all have the potential for creating process addictions. If going into an all-you-can-eat restaurant triggers that feeding frenzy energy, don't go in them when you're newly abstaining. If eating "dieting foods," such as cottage cheese, triggers your dieting mentality, pick other foods for the first few months. If *eating your favorite binge food* creates that rush, avoid them for a while. If *depriving yourself of your favorite binge food* creates more obsessional energy, plan a moderate serving in one of tomorrow's meals. If using dieting paraphernalia, such as measuring and weighing tools (for food or body), kicks in the control energy and obsession, don't use them. The disease will never want us to be honest, but if we do get rigorously honest, we will become aware of our own personal process addictions. We will become aware of what feeds our disease and what feeds our recovery.

If these process addiction/eating disorder enmeshments are not clearly understood nor properly prepared for, they will put the newly recovering person at risk for relapse. Discovering them and avoiding them can make early recovery saner and more stable.

In the following chapters, I hope to offer you some clarity about the disease and the beginning stages of recovery. In addition, this book should supply you with tools to permanently rid yourself of the obsessions, to expose the common pitfalls that breed relapse and to help you uncover the ways you've "*used*" your eating disorder for protection, manipulation, communication—to survive in the world. It will invite you to believe there is a way to live sanely and safely ***without*** an active eating disorder.

CHAPTER 2

WHY "NO RANDOM EATING"?

Random eating is the part of the disease that keeps us stuck in the feeding frenzy energy—the eating compulsion/obsession. Compulsive, impulsive, spontaneous, random eating is the first facet of an eating disorder to arrest. It will need a firm bottom line. The food and body image obsessions are equally important but usually they can't be clearly understood or adequately addressed when we are still randomly eating, dieting, restricting, grazing, bingeing, etc.

Because options can invite obsessions, giving up the option to eat randomly can bring freedom from the obsession to eat. Think about something you reserve the option to do but don't normally do, for example, keeping something that you find. What happens when you come across an article or money someone lost? If the article is something you want or need, then do you keep it? When the amount is several hundred dollars, then what? The struggle of deciding what to do and thinking, "should I or shouldn't I?" invites worry, upset and temporary obsession. If you don't have the option of keeping anything that isn't yours then the decision is simple and . . . no obsession! If you give up the option to eat in between meals, decisions are simpler and . . . no eating obsession!

If you can come to believe that you have an illness and that the way to arrest it is to not randomly eat, then what excuse or situation can ever justify not taking your "medicine" of no eating in between moderate meals? The slogan "three meals a day, nothing in between, **no matter what**" grants a great deal of freedom. Since 1974 I haven't found any situation, social or emotional, that required I eat in between meals!

In this society it's common to eat three meals a day, breakfast, lunch and dinner. Sometimes we have a day with just brunch and dinner, a two-meal day. If you have a health condition or lifestyle in which four meals would make more sense, eat four meals a day. (My personal experience is that four meals a day is harder emotionally and mentally . . . the disease has a chance for more manipulation, and therefore more relapse possibility.)

Remember, we need a bottom line definition of abstinence to arrest the disease. Be watchful of your motives; my suggestion is never **spontaneously** or **randomly** change the number of meals. Talk it over with someone who is supportive and understanding of your recovery. Remove the word *snack* from your vocabulary. A snack is usually just an accident with food, usually random eating. Don't save some food "just in case" of stress. Find new ways of dealing with stress reduction, ones that don't feed your disease.

It's usually impossible to find much clarity or stability in our recovery if we aren't abstaining from compulsive, impulsive, spontaneous, random eating. Commit yourself to abstinence, 100 percent of the time. Just as alcoholics aren't "perfect" because they're sober, we aren't perfect because we're abstinent, just as alcoholics **can** be sober 100 percent of the time, we can be abstinent 100 percent of the time from aberrant, addictive eating.

Don't mix up your definition of healthy eating with your definition of abstinence. If you have food allergies and/or food sensitivities, deciding whether or not you are currently eating them is a **separate** health issue.

Your definition of abstinence should be the bottom line needed to arrest your eating disorder. Make sure your definition addresses your eating problem history. If you have some process addictions, like vomiting or exercise purging, you might want to include a phrase in your definition that addresses those. If you have any non-narcotic substance addictions that you used to control your eating disorder, like laxatives or diuretics, you might want to address those by including a phrase that states a bottom line for those too. Write it down in black and white—make it as concrete as possible. There are some examples in the chapter, "What's Black & White & What's Grey?"

If you have now defined your abstinence and made a commitment to go to any length to honor it, you are ready to stay abstinent and to live abstinent from the compulsion and obsessions of an eating disorder. Anyone can diet for a brief time. Most of us have done it lots of times. The trick is to find tools that enable us to live without the obsession with control and without the obsessions with eating, food and body—without compulsive, random eating.

CHAPTER 3
DIETING MENTALITY

The dieting mentality is so ingrained in our thinking that the breadth and depth of it is amazing. Dieting usually increases the mental obsession to eat, the preoccupation with food and the focus on body image, which are, interestingly, the three primary eating disorder obsessions. The more focused and obsessed we become with "body sculpturing" and calorie restriction and/or elimination, the higher we measure our success. This insanity is common whether or not we have an eating disorder.

It's no wonder we are always looking for another new diet, another new way to regain control. Regaining control is what the "winners" do, right? No wonder we feel like failures in this society and no wonder the dieting industry is a multi-billion dollar business. **Sadly, everything about dieting feeds this disease.**

Facing our dieting mentality will be a critical ingredient in our recovery. It is one of the most important issues to address if we want to avoid relapsing. Many of the attitudes connected with dieting are so subtle that we aren't even aware of them. They are so familiar that we don't feel the urge to challenge, rethink or reject them. The dieting mentality can impact our whole outlook on life, influence major life decisions and daily minor choices. It can affect our relationship with others and with ourselves, destroy our peace of mind, but most of all, it can threaten our continuous recovery.

Exploring some of the most familiar expressions of the dieting mentality can help you begin to expose the danger of this cunning mindset. It will allow you to challenge, re-evaluate and redecide about these subtle beliefs that we have often hidden from ourselves. Here are some of the most common examples of this mentality:

- choosing foods or beverages for calorie content instead of nutritional value
- assigning value to self and others based on clothes size &/or body shape
- feeling "good" or "bad" based on calorie intake or food choices
- feeling shame for what we eat
- feeling shame for what we want to eat
- feeling shame for what we weigh
- feeling shame for what our body looks like
- believing the "right" combination of food and exercises will make us valuable
- believing there are "free" foods
- picking clothes to *hide* body size and shape
- picking clothes to *expose* body size and shape
- refusing social events or activities based on body image
- believing we should deprive ourselves of certain foods to be acceptable/OK
- living the "I'll start tomorrow, so today I'll..." mentality
- judging others' value by "looks"/body image
- deciding *our* value by "looks"/body image

Start to observe your thoughts. Begin to listen to the internal chatter and question your choices of food, clothes, friends, activities, etc. Try to avoid a quick rationalization. Become aware of the beliefs that you've been living by, very possibly without your adult self's conscious consent. Challenge any thoughts that tell you people are not OK based solely on body size and shape.

Haven't we gathered enough proof through the years that food choices and physical appearance don't accurately reflect kindness, courage, generosity, compassion, communication skills, ability for intimacy or interest in commitment? Yet, we were sometimes devastated and often repeatedly disappointed in our friends and lovers when we picked them with our eyes and not our hearts. Sometimes we have even blamed **our** appearance when we have been treated poorly, rejected or ignored.

I began challenging the dieting mentality by asking myself questions. "Do I want a relationship with someone who has picked me for my looks? Do I want my closest friendships to be based on external qualifications or internal qualities? Is exercise for my heart and soul or to influence my opinion and/or your opinion of me? Are thin people more competent, loving, disciplined, honest or safe?" Asking these questions began to allow me the option of redeciding about my beliefs.

I tried to notice commercials using the "taste test" concept to influence food buying. This subtle concept hides the belief that, "my tongue is the organ to make my health and nutrition decisions."

I tried to identify feelings of shame and to check whether their core was in my lack of understanding about my eating problem. Guilt says I made a mistake, shame says I am a mistake! When I chose to believe that eating disorders were an illness and not a moral issue, much of my shame began to fade and my self-forgiveness began to bloom.

If we continue to live by the dieting mentality, abstinence will continue to feel like a diet. We won't be able to move from the self-hate and moral judgment into the serenity of recovery unless we discard the dieting mentality. This dangerous mentality will eventually feed the attitude of "What's the use . . . It doesn't matter if I do, and it doesn't matter if I don't." This thinking **always** precedes a physical relapse.

Chapter 4

WHAT'S BLACK & WHITE AND WHAT'S GREY?

Having a "black and white" definition of abstinence means having a clear picture of when we're recovering and when we're not, knowing when we're abstaining and when we're not. If it all stays "grey" we will usually stay caught in the obsessive/compulsive cycle, the relapse cycle.

Therefore, one of our first tasks in recovery will be to find a "bottom line" for ourselves. If we find that bottom line, a statement that clearly defines abstinence, we will have found the black and white.

Using a black and white definition of abstinence will sound unacceptably restrictive in the beginning, but if we're serious about permanent relief, a bottom line will offer us freedom—real relief from our obsessive/compulsive relationship with food and eating.

In recovery from alcoholism, the need for continuous sobriety is a given; it gets the best results. Going on and off the wagon can be deadly for an alcoholic.

As with alcoholism, eating disorders need continuous abstinence to achieve the best recovery. When we're still attempting to control our eating and emotions with our on and off eating/dieting, we stay caught in the progressive, harmful effects of the illness. Stable emotions and stable weight will eventually show up when we commit ourselves to living the belief that no excuses can justify a break in continuous abstinence.

Here are some possible choices for a black and white definition of abstinence—a bottom line:

- no eating in between moderate meals, **no matter what**

- no eating in between moderate meals, no vomiting, **no matter what**
- no random eating in between moderate meals, **no matter what**
- no random eating in between moderate meals, no vomiting, **no matter what**
- no eating in between planned moderate meals
- moderate meals only, no random eating, no vomiting

If you also want to write out a definition of healthy eating and/or healthy nourishing so you're clear about the difference, it might be a very valuable assignment. Using this information, you can design guidelines for menu planning. But remember:

- a specific food plan is **not** abstinence *nor* is one required for abstinence
- there is no food craving that justifies a break in abstinence

You might want to follow the American Heart Association guidelines or the Pritikin Program guidelines most of time and then, when on a business trip or taking a vacation, you just simply make the best nutritional choices possible. Eating healthy 60-80 percent of the time is a goal within reach!

When we have our black and white definition of abstinence, we will discover grey areas that can also offer us much freedom. The grey areas can offer us the flexibility to live in this world and still recover from our eating disorder. Some examples of grey behavior are:

- Having only two meals in one day, brunch and dinner, when our day started mid-morning.
- Having juice or a cup of broth when there is more than a 6-hour period in between meals.

- Planning either a lunch or dinner of hot dog, popcorn, and soda when we go to a movie.
- Using a plate of hors d'oeuvres as our third meal at a social gathering.
- When traveling across several time zones, planning in a fourth meal.

This flexibility can be used to make continuous abstinence livable **but** it can also be abused to make abstinence difficult or shaky. *The grey is not good or bad.* Using our behavior with food and eating to define us as good or bad is an expression of the dieting mentality that is so subtle and cunning. Be sure and read the next chapter, "The Danger of Living in the Grey."

When we have a bottom line—a clear definition of abstinence we can live with 100 percent of the time—we can experience the comfortable knowledge that no matter what life has to offer, we can abstain, we can recover.

CHAPTER 5
THE DANGER OF LIVING IN THE GREY

Just as each of the examples of grey behavior can offer a tool for comfortable recovery, each one can be abused and lead to trouble. We can expect obsession to return if our motives for choosing grey behavior are based on a controlling, dieting mentality or on the "What can I get away with and still be in recovery?" mentality. When we begin to live in the grey, we slip into abusing flexibility—we begin to slide toward a physical relapse.

Look at the examples of grey behavior from the preceding chapter. If we begin to eat junky, chemical-laden, calorie-dense meals as the rule of thumb instead of the exception, our weight and sanity will be affected. If we justify a two-meal day regularly it will feed control and deprivation—the old dieting mentality. If we habitually choose caloric beverages such as smoothies, fruit juices and/or sodas, our weight will reflect it and our body image may become a relapse issue. When we consistently choose large meals, (what I call the high-end-of-moderate) we're looking for our old buddy food to be the answer to our pain or fear in life. *Again, we're stuck in the illusion that food, eating, or a certain weight will supply happiness, serenity or safety.*

Using the grey for flexibility and freedom is living in recovery. But abusing the grey is living in an emotional relapse and standing on the edge of physical relapse. It's just a matter of time before a full-blown physical relapse appears. *Physical relapse is always preceded by relapse thinking and increased grey behavior.*

With all of our grey area choices, we will need to examine our motives. We will need to ask ourselves, "Does this action or behavior feed the disease or does it feed the recovery?" If living in the recovery sounds hard, compare it to living in the disease. Remember, there is nothing so awful that a relapse can't make worse!

Chapter 6

RECEIVING THE OVEREATERS ANONYMOUS MESSAGE

Two thousand years ago, before epilepsy was viewed as an illness, people who had seizures were treated as if they were possessed by evil spirits and were condemned to live outside of society. These poor unfortunates were doomed to isolation, insanity and eventually death. Thankfully, we now know epilepsy is an illness; thankfully, the social stigma and bigotry today is nothing like the past.

Similarly, in the early 1900s, chronic alcoholics often lived outside of society and were also doomed to isolation, insanity and eventually death. Today there is an acknowledgement of alcoholism as an illness. Some research suggests that alcoholism has a biological predisposition.

Because of the leadership of Alcoholics Anonymous in the field of alcoholism recovery, many inpatient and outpatient programs have incorporated A.A.'s 12-Step solution in a multi-disciplinary approach to alcoholism treatment. A.A.'s 12-Step solution involves working your way, one step at a time, through a series of 12 Steps, moving on to the next one when you fully understand and have accomplished the task of the previous one.

In 1960, the newly formed Overeaters Anonymous adopted these 12 Steps of recovery from Alcoholics Anonymous, changing only the words "alcohol" and "alcoholic" to "food" and "compulsive overeater." O.A.'s 12 Steps are:

1. We admitted we were powerless over food—that our lives had become unmanageable.

2. Came to believe that a Power greater than ourselves could restore us to sanity.

3. Made a decision to turn our will and our lives over to the care of God, *as we understood Him.*

4. Made a searching and fearless moral inventory of ourselves.

5. Admitted to God, to ourselves and to another human being the exact nature of our wrongs.

6. Were entirely ready to have God remove all these defects of character.

7. Humbly asked Him to remove our shortcomings.

8. Made a list of all persons we had harmed, and became willing to make amends to them all.

9. Made direct amends to such people wherever possible, except when to do so would injure them or others.

10. Continued to take personal inventory and when we were wrong, promptly admitted it.

11. Sought through prayer and meditation to improve our conscious contact with God, *as we understood Him,* praying only for knowledge of His will for us and the power to carry that out.

12. Having had a spiritual awakening as the result of these steps, we tried to carry this message to compulsive overeaters and to practice these principles in all our affairs.

At first glance, the 12 Steps may appear to be religious in nature, but upon closer examination of their literature, the distinction between religious and spiritual will become evident. Their overall message is seasoned with a "take what you like and leave the rest" attitude, allowing atheists, agnostics and the devoutly religious all room to find their own path to recover.

The 12 Steps are best worked in the context of the 12-Step program, therefore, I will not be explaining how to work them.

The Overeaters Anonymous approach to eating disorders, the 12 Steps, and a supportive fellowship have proved immensely successful in addressing these cunning and baffling addictive diseases. Including O.A.'s message in a clinical/medical approach to dealing with eating disorders presents a powerful treatment plan.

Overeaters Anonymous literature tells us we have an illness that impacts our mind, body and spirit, and that willpower, emotional health and self-confidence are no defense against it. If we *could* have done better we *would* have done better.

None of us started a diet wanting to fail. None of us wanted the humiliation of gaining back all our weight plus more. None of us wanted to endure the social, emotional or physical consequences of obesity. None of us wanted the devastation of being discovered in the bathroom vomiting. None of us **gave** ourselves this disease, **but** at some point in our past we unconsciously began to perceive and design benefits from *using* our disease to deal with life.

O.A. invites us to believe that as a result of abstaining from compulsive overeating and living the spiritual principles reflected in the 12 Steps of O.A., we can find "a Power greater than ourselves" that can enable us to live free of the devastating effects of an eating disorder.

Just as alcoholics need continuous sobriety to recover, compulsive overeaters will need continuous abstinence. The book <u>Overeaters Anonymous</u> includes first-hand experiences in using the 12-Step recovery. It offers wonderful insight about the illness and the solution.

There is great news and great help in a 12-Step saying, "The 3 C's". By using the 3 C's slogan, "You didn't cause it, you can't control it and you can't cure it," we are invited to give up all our old blaming, condemning mentality. What a relief to finally resign from the task force of placing blame, on others or on ourselves. What a relief to know that although it can't be cured, there is a method for arresting it, that in fact, provides a "healing."

You can write or call Overeaters Anonymous World Service Office, P.O. Box 44020, Rio Rancho, New Mexico 87174-4020, 505-891-2664, and order their books and some basic information. You can also request the nearest O.A. contact in your local area.

CHAPTER 7
MODERATE IS MODERATE IS MODERATE

If there ever was a need to connect with our honesty and stop all denial, it's when we deal with the issue of what is moderate. This is not a disease that has included moderation of any kind, so developing a functional relationship with our honesty will be an absolute necessity.

The book <u>Alcoholics Anonymous</u>, in the first paragraph of chapter five, "How It Works," mentions **honesty** three times. It tells alcoholics that their chances of recovery are less than average unless they are capable ". . . of grasping and developing a manner of living which demands rigorous honesty." It also says, "There are those, too, who suffer from grave emotional and mental disorders, but many of them do recover if they have the capacity to be honest." It states that those who fail to recover are, "usually men and women who are constitutionally incapable of being honest with themselves."

Just as self-honesty is a key ingredient in arresting alcoholism, self-honesty is a primary tool in arresting an eating disorder. An active eating disorder will increase our denial about being unable to recognize moderate. But my experience as executive director of a residential center for women with eating disorders was, that even when a new resident was assigned the task of preparing and serving meals for their first time, they could accurately "guess" at moderate. They nervously thought they wouldn't be able to judge moderate, but when directed by a staff member to go ahead and make up one plate reflecting their guess at moderate and we would give them a "reality check," 99 percent of the time, they were right on target! My belief is that our honesty is usually there, it's just hidden behind the disease.

Honesty is one of the spiritual principles reflected in A.A.'s suggested recovery program. Probably the most critical one we will need to achieve abstinence and recovery. Honesty, moderate, abstinence and recovery are inseparable.

Moderate is an abstinence issue. When we begin to abstain, we begin to eat average, average in both in frequency and portions. What's average in our culture is three moderate meals a day. We have words for breakfast, lunch and dinner. We also have the word brunch, which labels the first meal of the day when it substitutes for lunch.

I believe moderate is a range. It has a high end and a middle range and a low end. It's not a target point and it's not exactly the same for everyone. Moderate is not a calorie count, but a portion size. If you put your hands together palms up, and then slightly cup them, right & left hand finger-tips touching, that's about the size of your stomach. What you eat at a meal, when chewed, should fit in your stomach. The reality of what is moderate is usually easier to identify than we want it to be.

Here are some of the suggestions I've heard over the years that help clarify "moderate."

- Moderate is more than "not enough" and less than "too much."
- Moderate is what you would serve yourself when you have company for dinner.
- Moderate doesn't feel stuffed.
- Moderate is average.
- Moderate is what you'd serve someone else recovering from an eating disorder.

I've seen the most success, meaning obsession-free eating, when we eat within the middle range of moderate most of the time and retain the option to eat at the low end or the high end of moderate from time to time. If we "live" at either the high end or the low end it usually feeds the disease, not the recovery. Eating consistently at either end usually feeds the disease **but** having the freedom to view moderate as a range can feed the recovery.

In addition to looking at the total quantity of a meal, it's equally important to be honest about what's an average or moderate serving of each type of food. For example, a meal consisting of ten ounces of steak and one cup of salad would not reflect a moderate serving of steak. A meal made up of two pieces of pie and two scoops of ice cream does not represent a moderate serving of sweets. A meal of all sweets is usually a relapse indicator. For a sane relationship with moderate, be willing to answer the question, "What's a moderate serving of what?"

Moderate is a relapse issue. I believe the most dangerous aspect of not predominantly eating in the middle range of moderate is that it sets the stage for relapse.

When we're eating at the low-end-of-moderate most of the time, it will trigger all those old diet mentality ideas and feelings. We will feel the elation of being "back" in control, feeling powerful, and having the "I finally got it under control this time" illusion. Eating consistently at the low end of the moderate range feeds false self-sufficiency and reinforces the denial of the disease. Also, consistent low-end-of-moderate eating will eventually lead to feeling deprived and hungry. This "dynamic duo" of deprivation and hunger can lead to a binge and trouble all the way around.

When we're eating at the high-end-of-moderate most of the time, we will feel all those old feelings—remorse, guilt, shame—the ones that usually accompanied a binge. It can lead to the "what's the use" relapse mentality. **Consistently eating at the high-end of the moderate usually means a higher than necessary body weight/size or weight gain.** Weight gain and/or a high-end-of-moderate body size will usually trigger our dieting mentality, food and calorie control obsession and body image obsession. All these consequences will block out growth and spiritual ideals and lead us back to our old relationship with food and body—to relapse.

Moderate is a health issue. When we consistently eat at the low-end-of-moderate or restrict and underfeed ourselves, not only can it trigger the dieting mentality, but we also run the risk of malnutrition and slowing down our metabolism. When we regularly eat at the high-end-of-moderate or consistently overfeed ourselves, we risk having an overweight problem, cardiovascular disease and many other degenerative diseases. Continually under or overfeeding ourselves will always block the sunlight of sanity.

I believe "eating only when we're hungry" is an idea to get rid of. Even when we're full, we can feel hungry. So don't worry about struggling to identify hunger, just eat your three moderate meals, **no matter what** and eventually, after three to nine months of continuous abstinence, become willing to identify **full**. It will reinforce honesty and it will support a healthy and healing relationship with our body.

If "what's moderate" remains a question that your honesty doesn't successfully answer, be willing to get a "reality check." Record your portions, including condiments, for seven to ten days, then label the meals as to whether you thought it was low, mid-range, or high moderate. Show the data to a sane, trusted friend—one who has no benefit in lying to you—or to your O.A. sponsor if you've already in O.A., or seek out a health professional who will discuss the moderate issue. Ask them for a reality check. Do not choose someone to answer the "what should I eat to lose weight?" question or the "how much should I eat to lose weight?" question, but someone to help answer the "what is a moderate serving for me?" dilemma. *When we consistently eat moderate, a moderate size body eventually shows up—without ever having to diet!*

Chapter 8
ONE MEAL AT A TIME, ONE DAY AT A TIME

If we use the 24-hour plan and just live today, not yesterday and not tomorrow, we can access a very powerful way to rid ourselves of the dieting mentality. And we *must* be rid of it to avoid a physical relapse.

Remember how we'd wake up Monday morning and promise today we will start our diet? Only to be unable to say no to a food we labeled as "taboo" offered at lunch? Or the times when we did temporarily achieve that goal weight—months of semi-starvation (with or without diet pills), months of cottage cheese, carrot sticks and **deprivation!** "Never again," we say, will we put the weight back on. We had sacrificed too much to allow that again!

Eventually, the memories of the daily suffering and deprivation faded and we found ourselves back to compulsively eating. In spite of our intentions, promises and insights, the outcome was almost always the same, disappointment, failure and self-hate. We seemed unable to live with dieting and unable to live without it, unable to live at our goal weight and unable to live without it.

Our friends and families have heard us commit to a new diet, a new weight loss plan, a new therapist, only to see us fail time and time again. Don't make another promise to *them*. Right now, commit to **yourself** not to eat until your next meal and continue reading this book.

If the desire to eat is really strong, divide the day into smaller parts. Decide not to eat for just the next hour. Take it just one hour at a time, one meal at a time. We can endure the temporary discomfort for just this hour, just this meal, just this day. Taking our abstinence one meal at a time will support a recovery mentality. It will challenge the dieting chatter.

If we start calorie swapping within a twenty-four hour period, it will trigger the dieting energy—the controlling, food manipulation insanity. Take it one meal at a time, one day at a time.

If any particular food is driving you crazy, plan a moderate serving in one of **tomorrow's** meals. One small piece of cake with tomorrow's dinner is a better plan than the "I can never have it again" mentality that sets you up for "going off" your diet/food plan or the midnight, "whole-cake" binge. Tomorrow, upon awaking, you can decide on your plan for the day. Your recovery can begin with one abstinent day.

We can put these dieting struggles behind us when we realize that *this* is the only day in which we can live. *This* is the only meal we can eat. It is much more realistic and comforting to say , "I'm not eating in between meals, just for today" than to live in the struggle, deprivation and controlling of dieting.

One of the ways I got through the day in the beginning of my abstinence was to take it just a few seconds or minutes at a time. If I was having trouble with the obsession to eat, I would focus my attention on my hand. I would refuse to move my hand (or body) toward food and I'd say to myself, "All I have to do is not move my hand right now, that's all, just not move, just for this one minute don't move." I'd repeat this single thought over and over, the moment would pass and, miraculously, the obsession would be gone. I found my mind had great difficulty holding two thoughts at the same time, so if the negative thought returned, I'd repeat the single-minded focus. The hour would pass and I'd make it to my next meal. Using this one tool, the day passed with no eating in between meals. Wow, the way I felt in the morning—no remorse, no guilt, no new self-hate.

I also learned by postponing the decision to act on a craving until tomorrow, I would often have changed my mind by the morning. But if I hadn't changed my mind, I would include a moderate serving of it at one of my moderate meals for that day. My willingness to go to any length to **not** eat in between meals, no matter what, began to have benefits. I discovered that no mental craving and/or no physical craving could justify compulsive eating or overeating! The phrase "no matter what" brought feelings of self-respect and self-esteem—of freedom and relief!

CHAPTER 9
DOES IT FEED THE DISEASE
OR DOES IT FEED THE RECOVERY?

This question may sound confusing but after a little thought a light usually goes on and we "get it." Since one of the goals of recovery is to increase serenity and decrease obsession, determining which thoughts and behaviors feed the disease and which thoughts and behaviors feed the recovery is critical. Challenge all activities/behavior choices with the question, "Does this feed the disease or does it feed the recovery?"

Picking at food while we cook often creates more and more eating frenzy energy, not recovery or calming energy. Activities such as baking goodies for holiday presents, can increase that obsession energy. Getting heavily focused on health, nutrition or exercise will also feed obsessional, dieting energy. So, don't place an unusual amount of time and attention on these activities in the beginning—hold off. We'll have plenty of time to deal with them when the recovery concepts of moderation and balance have become well established.

This question, simply reworded, can be used in all our daily living. "Does this activity or attitude increase my calmness or does it increase my anxiety?" "Does this choice support the positive direction I'm now going in, or does it encourage the old negative way?" "Does this action increase my self-respect or does it decrease my self-esteem?" "Will this take me toward full recovery or toward an active disease?" All of these variations pose the same question, "Am I choosing a life enriching or life depleting path?"

Here's a list of disease-calming actions:

• Serve moderate, eat moderate, no seconds.

- Restaurants often serve high-end-of-moderate meals, so a good rule of thumb is, eat 1/2 to 2/3 of what is served if you are a woman and 2/3 to 3/4 of the meal if you are a man.
- Never **redecide** about the portions or content once you begin eating—we definitely lose a healthy perspective after we begin a meal.
- Be aware of condiment abuse; use them sparingly.
- Excessive gum chewing or ice chewing in between meals leads to trouble— avoid it.
- Avoid meals that only consist of sweet-tasting foods.
- Don't binge on liquids to suppress the driving need to eat.
- Give up your membership in the clean-your-plate club.
- Be honest about salad bars and moderate fat intake (look at salad dressing and pasta salads' fat/oil content realistically).

These suggestions will be especially useful in the first year or two of recovery. Just as the alcoholic is better off in the first year of sobriety if he avoids hanging out in bars, the first year of your abstinence will be easier if you choose behavior that is disease calming.

Being willing to think before we act—to live at a conscious level—will not eliminate enjoyable spontaneity permanently. Up until now often our spontaneous reactions have not been enjoyable, but rather have been connected with that feeling of being out of control, resulting in failure. We have been used to stuffing our upset feelings with food or to blurting out our anger with hurtful words we later regret. What we need in the beginning of recovery is a new path and a new action. Pausing to answer this simple question, "Does it feed the disease or does it feed the recovery?" can be the beginning of a new peace, a new way of life.

CHAPTER 10
KEEPING IT SIMPLE

Don't complicate your eating disorder recovery. Too much analyzing can be paralyzing, especially in the beginning. Looking for **the** cause is nonproductive. We will eat when we're bored and when we're anxious, to celebrate a joyous occasion and to commemorate a sad affair. Because we have an eating disorder, we can justify eating over anything and everything, for every reason and no reason, when things are good and when things are bad.

Stay aware that the key words in my simple description of an eating disorder are "an **irrational** driving need to eat."

Although we have developed a pattern of *using* our disease to deal with life—and we will need to explore that history at some point in our recovery—keep in mind the disease can and will suggest/demand eating over anything, everything and nothing!

When any of the primary or secondary obsessions begin that internal chatter with us, confusion about what to do will also occur. Planning out our day, planning our meals, dressing for work or just getting ready to go into social situations can ignite relapse thinking—obsessional mind-chatter. In these times of confusion, simply "do what's in front of you." Take the next logical action, make the bed, go shower, write the report, make the phone call, drive home, read the paper, etc. Stop thinking, take a positive action and remember no random eating and no spontaneous meals!

Slogans are one of the most useful tools in confusing times. Here are some I've seen work. Most are 12-Step program slogans but several are mine.

- This too shall pass
- Do the foot work
- One day at a time
- K.I.S.S. (Keep it simple, stupid)
- Live and let live
- Stop analysis paralysis
- First things first
- Just for today
- Easy does it, but just do it
- It's only a meal
- Go with the flow
- Just do what's in front of you
- What's the loving thing to do?
- What's black & white & what's grey?
- Eat to nourish, not control
- Does it feed the recovery or does it feed the disease?
- If living in the recovery sounds hard, consider living in the disease

Taking one of these slogans and calmly repeating it over and over, sometimes while taking action, sometimes while remaining still, will often quiet a racing mind and stop the confusion.

When we commit ourselves to abstaining from compulsive eating one meal at a time, one day at a time, we've got a start. When we find a definition of abstinence that we can live with 100 percent of the time, we've got a chance for the obsession to eat to be removed. When we define healthy eating, understanding that it is not synonymous with abstinence, and attempt to eat healthy 60-75 percent of the time (that's probably higher than the average U.S. citizen), we've got a chance for the obsession with food to be removed. When we understand how to keep it simple, calmness and sanity can return.

CHAPTER 11

WATCH OUT FOR THE "PINK CLOUD"

You know the over-elation that goes with a successful diet? That feeling of finally regaining control as we experience a weight loss? That feeling that our eating problem is finally a thing of the past, that we will never lose control again? Sometimes the beginning of abstinence can feel similar to that. Things are going great and we feel normal . . . **Watch out!** Feeling normal or cured is a relapse indicator. A relapse into feeling we are cured, feeling we are cured of our old patterns and thoughts can lead to a physical relapse of random eating. Random eating leads to compulsive, out-of-control eating and weight gain, and eventually we relapse into repeated attempts to control—the old cycle.

I've often met people who, because they don't know I'm recovering from an eating disorder, think I'm a saint when they discover I don't eat in between meals, **no matter what** and I eat moderate, **no matter what!** To me it's simply understanding that I have an eating disorder, that it's an addictive disease and that my "medicine" of no random eating in between moderate meals allows me to live free of the devastating consequences!

It will be necessary to hang on to the understanding of the addictive disease concept. A.A. tells alcoholics that they "are like men who have lost their legs, they never grow new ones." We can learn from that statement. We need to learn to accept the permanency of the disease. Acknowledge to yourself that it's not a situation that can be defined as cured—only arrested, one day at a time.

When you affirm that the journey toward health is to live the recovery **just for today**, peaceful joy replaces the pink cloud of elation. We never "have it made," but we can have all the power we need to live just **this** day, sanely eat just **this one meal** by utilizing the 12 Steps and all the recovery tools.

CHAPTER 12
THE GREAT OBSESSION

Compulsive eaters have various obsessions—eating, food and body image are the primary ones. Most of us are familiar with the secondary ones—nutrition, exercise and health. The focus we place on these subjects is definitely immoderate!

I'm convinced though, that there is one "great obsession" that undermines every attempt to change. It usually sounds like:

If I get emotionally well enough . . .

If I get enough therpay . . .

If I get enough insight about me and my past . . .

If I get spiritual enough . . .

THEN I wll be a Normal Eater!

This delusion, which is usually kept just below the surface of conscious awareness, is very persistent. We are driven in our search to be "fixed"—if we find the right diet, if we find the right combination of healthy foods, if we find out what food we're allergic to and avoid it, if we find the right therapist, if we find the "thing" that happened in our past, understand it and heal it, we will be able to eat normally. We live with the secret hope of one day being fixed—being a normal eater.

Once we understand the nature of our illness and start recovery, we sometimes discover that we are frantically working the 12 Steps with the hope of being *cured*. But just as a little random drinking can lead to a binge for the alcoholic, a little random eating can lead to a binge, dieting, weight gain and relapse into obsession and compulsion.

We often wonder why therapy hasn't worked very well for us. Sometimes we hide the secret obsession to be "fixed" from ourselves. We hide it from the therapist. We search our past looking for a culprit. We try to find a person or situation to blame, something that could explain this insanity of eating beyond physical hunger.

Sometimes we find a tragedy that could explain this "quirk of character" and through understanding, forgiving and healing we secretly hope that now we will be like others, and simply eat to exist, not exist to eat. Disappointment hits when we discover that the information and processing didn't fix us; it didn't make us normal eaters.

When a recovering alcoholic uncovers memories of being molested by a neighbor or of being abused as a child, she usually doesn't have the hidden belief that *now* she will be a normal drinker. She finds a competent therapist and deals with the past memories so she can live a fuller life today. She has accepted her disease—she has let go of the idea that someday, somehow she will be a normal drinker.

After we have accepted our disease is when therapy really becomes beneficial. We've quit waiting to be fixed and commit ourselves to recovery. Once committed to abstinence, therapy is one of the most powerful tools in our recovery.

CHAPTER 13
SEEKING PROFESSIONAL HELP

Utilizing psychological or spiritual expertise is not in conflict with recovering from an addictive disease—an eating disorder, nor is it in conflict with working a 12-Step program. Just the opposite, it can greatly enrich our recovery. Refusing to accept a supportive hand from a professional helper can even be dangerous, an obstacle to recovery.

Unfortunately though, some of us have had a disappointing experience with a helping professional prior to arresting our eating disorder. When we begin to honestly look at our part in the therapeutic relationship, we have had to admit that we weren't always the easiest group to deal with. We sometimes omitted, lied or misled about our eating, dieting, exercising, etc. We didn't always follow instructions or suggestions. We often didn't fulfill our end of the relationship.

Our expectations were that we would be "fixed." We unconsciously waited for the wave of the wand to remove this despicable "defect." We talked and talked and waited for the magic to happen.

Now, armed with a new understanding about ourselves and the illness and a new respect for our own active role in our recovery, we can feel ready to utilize good professional help. We can give up the Great Obsession that we will someday get the *right* therapist or *enough* counseling to make us normal eaters. We can get on with real change and growth and let go of the old delusions.

Locating a therapist who is experienced in "codependency" issues will be of immense value. A simple definition of codependency is continuing to react from unresolved childhood/adolescent experiences instead of living from conscious, deliberate beliefs and actions that enrich our life.

The more dysfunctional our childhood environment and/or our primary caretakers, probably the more we have used our disease to help us cope with life, and consequently the more entwined our eating disorder and codependency issues will be.

Even though the disease will tell us to eat over anything, everything and nothing, *how we used our disease* to protect, manipulate, set boundaries (emotional, intellectual, physical and sexual) and avoid feelings and life in general, will be critical information if we want to live a functional, serene life. Discovering and designing new ways to protect ourselves, setting healthy boundaries and making peace with our history will offer us a life free of **needing** our disease. A codependency expert will usually have the insights and tools necessary to help us recover, recover from the eating disorder, codependency enmeshment.

Once we have an understanding of the recovery process and an awareness of our role in that process, we can begin to accept responsibility for our paths in life. We can begin to gracefully accept the guiding and supportive role professionals can offer us.

CHAPTER 14
INSTITUTIONAL MENTALITY

Like the dieting mentality, the institutional mentality is incredibly subtle, only this one isn't openly talked about, easily identified or exposed. Potentially, it can contaminate your relationship with recovery in general, and with treatment programs or treatment professionals, specifically.

Institutional mentality often gets spawned by the dieting mentality. We start looking for that outside "fix" or "fixer." The search for the newest diet, diet doctor or diet center can be the start of this powerful mind-set. When we're seduced by the words *easy, painless* and *quick,*— very commonly, the adjectives that the dieting industry uses to advertise— we are vulnerable to the institutional mentality.

Instinctively, we know we need a "Power greater that ourselves" but unfortunately, when we've adopted the institutional mentality, we begin to look for someone or something to place on a pedestal, something to assume responsibility for getting us fixed and keeping us safe.

If our eating disorder has progressed enough for us to start down the therapeutic path, the outpatient role is fertile ground for this dangerous mind-set. Unconsciously, we begin to assume the institutional mentality posture in the therapeutic setting: "I'm hopelessly defective and have no answers, **you** have the answers, the hope and the cure, please wave your magic wand over me."

If we take on such a passive posture, we will usually only "do good" for a while. When it seems like they've put the magic wand down, we often crash in depression and relapse. Eventually though, we begin our search for the next fix/fixer.

The person who has this cunning mentality in the extreme, usually has a history of years of therapy, "therapist hopping" and/or numerous hospitalizations, sometimes bingeing, vomiting and/or starving right through the hospital stays. The inpatient role, with all of its potential for healing and growing, can covertly feed this damaging mentality.

Not all compulsive eaters with this mentality progress to the extremes I've mentioned, but most of us have some hint of it. I've listed below some the most common mental postures that reflect an institutional mentality.

- I can't be trusted on my own
- The "right" structure will control me
- I feel "less-than" in all primary relationships
- Where can I go to re-group and be taken care of?
- I believe my recovery/existence is contingent upon maintaining my relationship with this person or facility
- I need you to give me *the* answers
- This is too hard, I need a place to rest (again)
- I will give them what I think they want, even if I lose me
- I can't trust my intuition or my "heart"
- Something outside of me should/could make me OK/ acceptable
- If I show you I'm trying, you won't abandon me

The institutional mentality will set us up to turn our will, and sometimes our lives, over to a person or a place. Letting a facility or institution help us help ourselves is great, but giving up a responsible posture for very long will usually feed the disease and a relapse, not recovery. If you're going to benefit from any professional setting and/or help, you'll need to be aware of the individual subtleties of your institutional mentality.

Even utilizing Overeaters Anonymous can be detrimental, if you look to a "program sponsor" as the newest fixer, or expect that simply sitting in an O.A. meeting will "abstain" you. Be watchful of the "If I do service and work the Steps, then one day I'll start abstaining—painlessly" concept.

Be willing to expose even the slightest hint of this mentality. Challenge these erroneous assumptions that support your feelings of being untrustworthy, unworthy or impotent. Be willing to find a supporter who encourages you to abstain, no matter what, to find your own answers and who celebrates your individually. Don't settle for anything less than a sponsor/supporter who insists you find a "God concept" you can do business with, a Higher Power that is the essence of your being, one that you can trust to love and care for you unconditionally. Seek a therapist and institutions that have a clarity about codependency and who refuse to feed the institutional mentality. Commit yourself to following a path that invites wholeness.

Recovery will be the hardest thing you'll ever do, but the 12-Step solution is designed to confront all of our old ideas and beliefs and guide and support us through the process of acquiring new ones, ones that foster and nurture a new way of living, feeling and thinking.

CHAPTER 15
WHAT ABOUT EXERCISE?

For some of you this is probably one of the first chapters you wanted to read, and others would prefer to skip the whole subject. No matter which extreme you relate to, it's definitely a subject we all need to deal with.

As with our eating, we probably don't have a healthy relationship with moderate exercise either. Often we're dominated by the dieting mentality of, "It's all or nothing" and "Anything worth doing is worth doing perfectly!" For some of us the bingeing mentality says to us, "If some is good, more is better." These old ideas have to be smashed. Whether you come from the exercise extreme of "body sculpturing" (with or without calorie purging) or you come from the "Why sit down when you can lie down," mentality, a new attitude and balance is needed. We're looking for moderate here—a subject with which we rarely have a passing acquaintance.

Since abstinence comes from a surrendered, non-controlling attitude, we'll want to use that same emotional posture when discovering our moderate range in exercising. Abstinence is based on love, love of self and love of life. It often doesn't feel that way in the beginning, but to pick a path of recovery is to pick life.

You can grow to enjoy exercise and love your body. Gently inviting your body to stretch, move and bend can be a welcome gift. I believe exercise, when done properly, brings enjoyable stiffness, not pain. It brings us increased energy, not depletion.

Therefore, finding out how to correctly begin an exercise regime is the key to a successful relationship with exercise. Some beginning suggestions for the compulsive **under-exerciser** are:

- Check with your favorite health professional—if they can't make some recommendations, ask for a referral.

- Get an "exercise sponsor"—someone who'll help keep you honest and sane in your choices, someone who's been successful at moderate exercising.

- Walk—start slow and with short distances, be willing to gradually increase, and learn how to find your target heart range.

- Spend one whole day keeping your focus on your posture— lovingly correcting it when you discover slumping.

- Purchase a couple of exercise books currently on the best seller list—pore over them, take notes and review the notes with your exercise sponsor or health professional (I loved Norman Cousins' book, The Healing Heart).

- Check out a local health club—ask about the background and training of the person representing the club, connect with the resident expert.

If exercise abuse has been part of your history, keep your eyes, ears and mind wide open. Exercise abuse is usually connected with body image issues and that's a number one relapse problem. If you're also an athlete, the need to search your motives at all times is paramount!

Some beginning suggestions for the compulsive **over-exerciser** are:

- Walk—build up to a swift pace but keep within your target heart range.

- Get an "exercise sponsor"—someone who'll support a sane and honest perspective, someone who has found freedom from compulsive exercising.

- Be willing to examine your motives about your sports involvement.

- Include a weekly meditation that focuses on

acknowledgement and recognition of the value of some of your major organs—heart, liver, stomach, intestines, muscles, skin, etc.—a quiet "thank you" to all for their past performances.

- Set up a weekly plan that includes a range, such as, "I will run 10 to 15 miles a week." Go over it with your sponsor or health expert and make a commitment to discuss it, *before* you exceed your top range.

Gradually returning to exercise purging can be a subtle, insidious process, an "accident" you don't need. You'll need the support of those who can help you recognize the red flag of relapse.

If you fall into the **moderate exerciser** category but exercise out of fear and resentment, some suggestions are:

- Make a list of reasons you exercise—fear of what, resentment of who and what. Look for the beliefs behind the "whys." The following paragraph offers an example of how to challenge the belief. By exploring the underlying beliefs, you will have a choice. You will get to decide if you want to continue to act as if you believe the old ideas.

Reason: "I exercise because I hate my big thighs." Belief behind: "I'll be more valued by myself and others if my body shape is a certain way or size." Challenge: "Do I value others because of their looks or because of their loving qualities?" "Do I value youth at the exclusion of wisdom?" "Do I want to be with someone who values me primarily for my looks?"

- Take the spiritual principle of love and place it in your heart, and when deciding about exercise, ask "What would love do?"

CHAPTER 16
EAT TO NOURISH, NOT CONTROL

There have been so many subtle ways we have attempted to control our food, our eating and our body size; subtleties in our thinking and in our actions. After years of attempting to control our eating and weight, the concept of simply nourishing ourselves is a difficult one, to say the least.

We chose foods (or drinks) for their caloric value instead of their nutritional value. We used the "taste test" philosophy to pick a food. We acted as if the tongue were the organ to make our health decisions. Just because our tongues can't tell the difference between a real strawberry and ethyl-3-methyl-3-phenylplycidate (a common strawberry flavoring), we ignored the fact that our bodies can!

We drank non-caloric beverages to quiet the "driving need to eat," silently resigned to the white-knuckling posture of avoiding calories at any cost. We ignored the notion that we could be polluting our body with additives and preservatives.

When we surrender and give up controlling, we have begun to accept the fact that we have an illness. As we let go of the attempts to control, we can spontaneously move into acceptance of the disease **and** the commitment to recovery.

We intuitively sense recovery means to nourish our body, mind and spirit. But when we start to nourish our body, we struggle to separate the old thinking from the new, the unhealthy from the healthy, the dieting from the abstaining.

Almost everything feels like control energy when we start to focus on and change our food choices; it feels like dieting. We unconsciously use the calorie count and taste test criteria and ponder why this doesn't feel like recovery.

When we begin to eat to nourish and not to control, we can find relief. When we begin to make our menu decisions coming from love, courage and surrender we begin to feel the recovery.

I want to offer some suggestions on how to build a healthier relationship with your body.

- Act as if you were designing a menu for someone recuperating from a serious illness. (You are!)
- Start to acknowledge and recognize the language of the body: rashes, gas, aches and pains, indigestion, fatigue, etc. (the body is a non-English- speaking entity.)
- Place the spiritual ideal of love in your heart when making health/food decisions. Answer the question, "What would love choose?"
- Work the Twelve Steps of Overeaters Anonymous. Be willing to make **direct** amends to your body (and organs) by abstaining.

Remember, none of these work very well if we don't consistently and clearly use the intent or energy of love and respect to take action. But sometimes being motivated by love is impossible, for one reason or another. So by remembering the pain of doing it the old way can be helpful. Avoidance of the pain of an active addiction can often be more motivating than self-love . . . but keep attempting to act from love, not pain.

With this new mind set, we can begin to seek additional nutritional information. Check the American Heart Association and the National

Cancer Institute's nutritional guidelines. Purchase a couple of the best selling books on nutrition. Two of my favorites are <u>Jane Brody's Nutrition Book</u> and <u>The Healing Heart</u> by Norman Cousins.

Come up with a working definition of healthy eating. Individualize it for you. Listen to your body. If strawberries give you a rash, omit them from your menus. Here are my guidelines for healthy eating:

- low animal protein
- low fats
- low salt
- low dairy products
- low sugar
- low processed foods
- low chemical-laden foods
- high fiber
- high complex carbohydrates
- high fresh fruit and vegetables

My definition of healthy eating came from various sources, including my body. I try to achieve my goal of healthy eating 75 percent of the time. When I'm traveling, I can't check the chemical content of airline food or restaurant food; I just "go with the flow." In reality, we do have the opportunity to choose the quality of our meals between 60-80 percent of the time.

Here are some nutritional tips. They're "flip," but easy to remember.

- When reading labels, if you can't pronounce it, don't eat it.
- Don't embalm yourself ahead of time.
- If it has a longer life span than you, don't eat it.
- Your tongue isn't the organ to make your health decisions.

- Moderate is a health issue.
- "Whole foods tend to produce whole cells and whole cells tend to produce whole bodies."

Living by spiritual ideals in recovery isn't easy and it certainly isn't clear at the start. Just staying away from that first compulsive bite in between meals is often the only thing we can do in the first few months. But as we begin abstaining and working the 12 Steps, we find some relief from the insanity of random eating. Self-respect and self-love begin to grow. When these increase, the ability to eat to nourish will increase.

In times of confusion or indecision, answering these important questions will help us sort through our struggle and find the relief of calm decision.

- Is this choice based on body sculpturing or body nourishing?
- Does it feed the disease or does it feed the recovery?
- What would "love" do/choose?

Remember, nourishing comes from an entirely different mind-set than dieting. For us, it comes from the spiritual principles of *acceptance* of our disease, *respect* of the disease, *honesty* about moderate and *love* of body and organs.

CHAPTER 17
MAINTENANCE: WHAT A CONCEPT!

I've seen people start abstaining (no eating in between meals), grab hold of a weight-loss food plan and follow it. They target a goal weight, feel excited, eat only certain foods, in certain portions and watch to see the weight come off—sounds like a diet, looks like a diet, feels like a diet. That's exactly how I started abstaining—with both dieting actions and dieting mentality. **But we don't have to start abstaining by going on one more weight-loss, weight-control diet. We can do it differently.**

We don't need to follow a weight-control diet when we start abstaining. We can start abstaining from compulsive overeating by going to any lengths to not eat in between three **moderate** meals a day. Miraculously and most of the time, when we eat only moderate meals, the "right" body will show up. Maybe not the body we'd pick, but the one nature has given us, the one we're supposed to love, cherish and accept.

Granted, many of us have damaged our metabolisms and sometimes there may be a health condition that requires a **therapeutic** diet, but arresting an eating disorder by abstaining is not synonymous with following a certain therapeutic diet.

When we begin to deal with a stable maintenance weight, honesty and clarity of mind is a vital ingredient. *Notice I used the words maintenance weight, not goal weight.* We will need **honesty** to acknowledge a moderate portion of food and a moderate meal. We need a clear mind to acknowledge the wide array of body sizes and shapes that fall in an average range category. We need enough honesty and willingness to get on a scale and see what it says when we continuously abstain by eating three moderate meals a day.

A problem arises when we have picked a goal weight. We say, "Look what I have given up!" and demand that we are rewarded with the body and the number on the scale we want. My experience and observation is that this demand can create relapse attitudes and behavior. Often we've picked the weight we were when we were fifteen years old or sometimes we've picked the number off a chart. In any case, we often end up withholding acceptance of our bodies and staying in the beginning stage of recovery by controlling our food and meals to get the goal weight we want.

Our unresolved body image issues will always rear their ugly heads when we address maintenance, **but resolving maintenance issues are the key to long term recovery.** If we never reach a normal weight range, if we never accept our body or weight, if we consistently eat at the high-end-of-moderate or the low-end-of-moderate, we will probably continue to struggle with primary and secondary obsessions. If we continue the struggle, we will stay relapse prone.

Dealing with maintenance in a honest, straight forward manner, is a very necessary step in long term recovery. Avoiding the scale is as much of a pitfall as relentlessly pursuing a goal weight. Because we have abused the scale, often making it a god that reflects our value and good or bad performance, we might tend to avoid the scale. But it will be important for us to look that erroneous belief right square in the eye and challenge it. We will need to develop a functional relationship with the scale—neither avoiding it nor serving it. Our value is not based on our looks or our body size. We all have innate value. Our value isn't higher because we're thinner or younger or taller or older or shorter or blonder or tanner. We don't have to deny that these societal beliefs exist, but **we** don't have to live by all of them either.

The scale can honestly reflect trends—a trend toward weight gain, a trend toward weight loss and a stability trend. It's information that can encourage us to keep our heads out of the sand. It's information that can help us avoid a slow slide into physical relapse. This data gathering process doesn't necessarily demand action. We must ask ourselves the following questions to utilize the information from the scale.

1. Am I abstaining 100 percent of the time?
2. Am I eating healthy 60 to 75 percent of the time?
3. Do I have a health condition that might be affecting my metabolism or weight?

Answering these questions implies willingness, honesty and clarity. It means you have a definition of abstinence and a separate definition of healthy eating. Usually the last question is difficult to answer in the first three to nine months of abstinence because our health has often been negatively impacted by our eating disorder. Since there is a good possibility that many of our disease-related health conditions will decrease or disappear with continuous abstinence, it might be best to wait for a minimum of three months of abstinence to answer question number three. (If your weight isn't moving toward a moderate range by nine months, it is definitely time to look at health problems.)

If you're underweight or in a moderate body size range, getting on the scale once or twice a month for the first six months of abstinence is plenty. If you are overweight, getting on the scale once or twice a month is also probably enough. If you have moved into a maintenance range, weighing once a week or every other week is appropriate. When you've noticed you're staying in a range of about three pounds up and three pounds down for about six months, that sounds like maintenance.

Bigger fluctuations might have a message for you. Don't look the other way. It could be either too many high-end-of-moderate meals, too many junky meals, a health condition such as menopause (or simply aging) or a health problem. Be honest and look.

One woman I know took a week and simply recorded how often she ate high-end-of-moderate meals. Her results showed about 50 percent of the time. That gave her the information she needed to explain her high-end-of-moderate body size. She brought the percentage down to about 25 percent and felt better physically, emotionally and spiritually and several pounds dropped off.

When you're ready to address the scale/weight issue, make sure you plan it—don't spontaneously weigh. Have a regularly scheduled morning to weigh, write out what your meals are going to be for the day so there's no chance for emotional manipulation at meal time and plan to call your sponsor or a support team member immediately after getting off the scale. Whatever body image issues that get activated when you weigh, you'll have someone to offer you a reality check about fat/thin, good/bad, and less-than/better-than. In the past, the scale gave us permission to be OK or condemned us to despicable, so a sane dose of reality will keep us from moving into physical relapse.

One young woman who had starved and purged her way down to 82 pounds, vowed to kill herself if she ever reached 100. But after continuously abstaining and working the 12 Steps, when she actually went over 100 (at about nine months of abstinence), she had enough freedom from the insanity of the disease to stay committed to her path of recovery.

She leveled out at about 106 for about four months and then her weight went up to 116. The increase happened in about a two month time period. She stayed abstinent and tried to realistically look at what changes had been going on with her food choices—quantity, as well as quality.

She had had a residential change, was eating junkier food and at the high-end-of-moderate more often. She looked at the fact that she had started to seek comfort and solace from the larger meals. She focused more consciously on the spiritual principles of *honesty, courage and surrender.* She returned to the quantity and quality of food she had been eating during the first year of her recovery.

By addressing these relapse indicators, she experienced the reality of working at her recovery. Over the next few months the extra ten pounds slowly melted away. When her weight was once again stable, what she talked about most was how she discovered a real liking for her body and finally a real enjoyment of the 106 pound body that she presently has.

My personal experience was that I went 15 lbs. **under** my goal weight. **I** decided what I should weigh—I picked a goal weight. **(Isn't it interesting that we don't have a *goal height* but we think we should have a goal weight?)** I am about 5'9 1/2" tall and weighed about 160 lbs. when I started abstaining. I thought 135 lbs. sounded like a good weight to be. I picked a weight-loss food plan similar to several around at the time (1974), a high protein, fruit and vegetables, no refined or complex carbohydrates. When I reached the goal weight I had picked for myself, I began increasing the portions on my food plan, but my weight continued to drop. I was encouraged to again increase the portions. When I went under my goal weight that was OK, but when I went 10 lbs. under, I was getting concerned and feeling ugly. A "rack of bones" was the way I thought of myself. Additionally, I soon discovered that these highest of the high-end-of-moderate meals triggered old, old feelings—feelings of remorse, guilt and self-loathing.

When I went more than 10 lbs. under, I decided to go off that food plan and eat moderate portions of more calorie dense food—**to only have healthy eating guidelines, not a food plan.** I decided to eat moderate portions of whatever restaurants or people served and to include complex and refined carbohydrates in my menu planning. I let go of banning foods, of labeling good foods/bad foods.

My weight leveled out at about 120 lbs., a couple of pounds up or a couple of pounds down, but pretty much 120 lbs. I felt unattractive and skinny. Acceptance was my problem and eventually, my answer. I tried to find people to talk to who could help me find that acceptance, but nobody seemed to relate to my particular situation.

One evening I was having coffee with a couple of recovering women friends. One of them was having a similar problem—she was 15 lbs. over the weight she wanted to be at. I thought she looked great but she was baffled as to why she hadn't reached the weight she wanted. She said, "I know I'm abstaining and I know I eat healthy, so I guess this is what God wants me to look like." Bingo, I had my answer!

I looked at the fact that nature had given me a body similar to my birth-father's family—thin and tall, not my mom's side of the family, which was medium height and voluptuous. I had tons of energy and hadn't been sick since I started abstaining, so I became willing to accept myself as I was. I started seeing myself in more realistic terms. I started picking clothes that complimented my body size and shape. I started feeling attractive.

This process for me took about six months at the same weight. My suggestion is to get the support from others and start on the path of honesty and acceptance. Be willing to abstain, no matter what. Be willing to eat moderate portions and moderate meals, no matter what. Be willing to weigh yourself regularly. Be willing to get honest about healthy eating. Be willing to get a reality check if you're not sure what's moderate or what's healthy eating. Ask another recovering, maintaining compulsive overeater's opinion. Read some nutrition books and get the American Heart Association guidelines. Be willing to honestly look at your beliefs about body size/shape/value—at your beliefs about "looks." Seek answers to your past and your pain. There are many good health professionals and many good therapists; be willing to seek their help.

We have blamed our weight and bodies for our situations. We have used our overweight, underweight and our "I'm not good enough" mentality to protect us from life and to stop us from living. We don't have to any more. There are answers and they will be found in the seeking.

The difference between weight controlling and eating disorder recovery is in our hearts and our attitudes. If you videotaped a person dieting and you videotaped a person abstaining, they might look very similar. **But the attitude in long-term abstinence has to do with freedom,** *not deprivation,* **a way of life,** *not temporary measures,* and **serenity with food, eating and body image,** *not obsession.*

CHAPTER 18
SURRENDER TO WIN. . . PARDON ME?

Who would have thought that by giving up the fight, we begin to win? My heart knew if I chose to continue the fight at all, I'd lose. But I thought if I didn't attempt to regain control, I'd be doomed to the consequences of being out-of-control. My mind struggled to make sense of the 12-Step phrase, "surrender to win."

I soon discovered that to surrender doesn't mean compliance, where we passively give up. It means to surrender and let go of the idea that we will ever be normal eaters and to put all of our energy and intelligence into arresting this lifelong illness.

I realized that I wouldn't fight **or deny** having diarrhea or epilepsy. That could be a humiliating or possibly a deadly pretense. Instead, I would definitely take steps to make my situation as safe and as comfortable as possible. I'd try to learn as much as I could about the condition, and I'd try to find out what action/inactions might facilitate the recovery. I'd want to learn to live in a way that arrests the illness, the things that keep it in remission.

When it comes to our eating problem, though, we don't immediately respond with the same compassion. We usually respond with a moral self-judgment, such as, "If I just had more willpower, I wouldn't be doing this" or "If I was a better person, a stronger person, I wouldn't be having this problem." Although not accurate assumptions, these are probably average replies.

Thankfully, we eventually experience severe exhaustion trying to use sheer willpower to control it. Exhaustion will often make us open to a new idea, a new way of looking at things—like the idea that it may not be a moral issue, that it might be an illness. In Alcoholics Anonymous, this exhaustion mixed with a little willingness to change ideas and actions is called "hitting a bottom." It might sound negative, but after you hit the bottom, you can start up again, up toward full recovery.

But still, many of us will be annoyed by O.A.'s use of the word "powerless." We'll feel we must reject the *powerless* concept to maintain a sense of competency about our life. The way I re-interpreted it was by using the example of my height. Even though in reality I can't change my height I don't experience a loss of power or competency based on that variable. In fact, if I had a *goal height* as an adult and spent time and energy obsessively focused on trying to achieve it, people would probably worry for my mental and physical health. If I was using my willpower to change my height, I would be a dismal, frustrated failure. But if I finally accepted my adult physical height, I would experience a return of sanity. By simply re-framing the idea it finally became palatable.

CHAPTER 19
CHANGING OLD ROUTINES

We've tried every imaginable way to hang on to our *old behavior* while trying to change our *thoughts and thinking*. We've tried every imaginable way to hang on to our old thinking while trying to change our behavior. These attempts usually reflect a faulty attitude that says half measures will produce whole, complete change.

The need to change that attitude is critical if we're serious about arresting this illness. There are two phrases that really help simplify this process. Make them your mantra for the first year of recovery: *act as if* and *fake it till you make it.*

Act as if you *believe* there is a Higher Power that will help you with your eating. Act as if 100 percent of you *wants* to let go of the food obsession (even when it's only 49 percent). Act as if you *deserve* sane living and healthy relationships. Act as if you *love* yourself. Don't stay in the rut of "I can't." Take action reflecting "I can."

Don't wait for the **feelings** of commitment, value or love to appear *before* you take recovery action. If we wait for those feelings to appear before we initiate action, we might wait forever. I never woke up one morning and said, "Hurray, today is the day I'm going to change everything about me, my old ideas and my old beliefs!" But I did wake up many mornings engulfed in shame and guilt, dreading the day before me, with no hope for real change and wondering how I could go on living this way, day after day. I'd promise myself that today would be different, never really believing it, and I'd get up and try one more time to do the same old things, hoping to get different results.

My disappointment and desperation were incredibly valuable

when I started to recover. They made me teachable, open and willing to let go of my old ways of acting and thinking.

Take the attitude and action of a person you would like to be. Use the "fake it 'till you make it" mentality. In the beginning of my recovery, I came up with a list of women I admired and in times of confusion I would say to myself, "What would Marjorie (or Sharon or Carol or Pat) do?" Asking that question, I always came up with an *attitude and action* that reflected someone who was loving, wise and tolerant of herself and others.

If the eating-frenzy energy kicks in, our blinders can really snap into place and we feel driven to *eat.* Just know you, **don't have to act on it**, and by taking an opposite, loving action, that driving need to eat dissipates rapidly. Change your location and/or redirect your attention. Go into another room or take a walk or make a phone call. Grab an inspirational book (or article) and take a reading break or repeat an affirmation (or favorite prayer) over and over. You'll discover the new action brings new self-worth and the feeding-frenzy energy will eventually change into simple thoughts about eating that we assign less and less importance to.

I want to share some ideas of things to change in the beginning. Remember, old behaviors lead to old thoughts and old thoughts lead to old behavior, while new behaviors can lead to new thoughts and feelings and new ideas can lead to new behavior.

- eliminate the option of seconds
- sit down to eat
- use a cloth napkin instead of a paper napkin
- use an attractive place mat
- don't eat while watching TV
- set the table as if you are having important guests
- serve and eat on glass, not plastic

- brush your teeth after each meal
- slow your eating down, chew and taste
- discover moderate: weigh and measure your food for 10 days (longer than 10 days will usually feed control, dieting energy)
- serve moderate, eat moderate
- don't bring home leftovers from restaurants
- begin a meal with a prayer of gratitude
- read an inspirational thought each morning and night
- wear clothes that fit
- cultivate an attitude of gratitude
- read literature daily that supports new ideas
- drive a different route to work
- try a new hair style

Break old routines. The quote **"We don't *think* our way into sane living, we *live* our way into sane thinking,"** is the ultimate truth for us.

CHAPTER 20
FIRST THINGS FIRST

This simple slogan is one that can keep us reminded of the priority to abstain, no matter what. In recovery from an eating disorder, abstinence will be a matter of the utmost importance, a matter of emotional, spiritual and physical survival.

This disease has been known to contribute to early death in various ways. But don't underestimate its power to remove the **quality** of life long before it might become life threatening.

Since random, compulsive eating/starving can activate the illness, we must be willing to take whatever action (or inaction) necessary to abstain, *and* whatever steps are necessary to make abstinence comfortable.

Committing ourselves to the priority of abstinence might bring up the question, "Does this mean I'm supposed to rank abstinence above other health issues, family, job, or friends?" When we are active in our disease, we are often powerless to honor other health conditions, as well as these important facets of life. Therefore, if we allow the disease to go unarrested, we might be at risk to lose family, job, health or friends.

When we finally understand and fully accept that our eating disorder is a potentially life-threatening disease, we can begin to address our eating disorder recovery and other health issues as equals. If you have another serious illness, you don't have to rank one higher or lower than the other, nor view the treatment or recovery as incompatible.

Abstaining doesn't imply perfection any more than sobriety implies that the alcoholic is now perfect. It's a matter of recovery and survival. Keep this perspective, abstinence can be done 100 percent of the time. Because we can admit we have this illness 100 percent of the time, continuous abstinence will reflect acceptance and respect. That's the goal, not perfection.

Once we make our abstinence a top priority, we can continue to benefit from the "First Things First" saying. We can use it as a tool to prioritize our everyday activities. At times, deciding between returning phone calls and taking a shower can create mental confusion. These mental dilemmas can lead to frustration and disappointment if we don't solve the prioritizing problem. Ask yourself, "How important is it?" and then arrange tasks and obligations based on your answers. Remember, when you're newly abstaining, it's best to keep your schedule relatively loose and your plans flexible.

As we continue to use the affirmation of "First Things First" on a daily basis, control and perfectionism will begin to dissipate. The priorities of recovery and a healthy perspective can bring an orderliness to our lives, and a peacefulness we have long yearned for.

CHAPTER 21

H.A.L.T. (HUNGRY, ANGRY, LONELY, TIRED)

For a stable recovery, there are at least four dangerous conditions which we must watch out for: hungry, angry, lonely or tired. Too much of any of these four will indicate our need to "HALT." When we get a large dose of any part of H.A.L.T., we will be at risk for relapse. In this precarious spot, we can lose our clarity and start moving toward the "what's the use" mentality.

In the beginning of our recovery, we will be very vulnerable to old ways of thinking and behaving. New information, tools and insights will only be as valuable as our willingness. And unfortunately, our willingness will suffer or lessen if any facet of H.A.L.T. puts us in that vulnerable state.

Not getting too hungry probably already makes sense. We've all experienced the set-up of small, restrictive meals. They simply scream for overeating. So for safety and sanity, commit to eating in the middle range of moderate. Not the high-end, not the low-end—just an average size meal. The disease will try to tell you you don't know what moderate is, but in reality, we do. I believe the honesty is there, we just aren't used to honoring it or recognizing it.

If you do find yourself in a situation where you're feeling too hungry by meal time, you will probably notice that you lose your clarity about what's moderate. That's when you might make a call to someone who's an understanding person, one who can discuss portion size honestly, or you might have some juice and relax a few minutes so you're not making portion size decisions without your "recovery clarity."

Not getting too angry will also be important. We have sometimes used anger at others, expressed or unexpressed, to justify a binge, break a diet or set off a starvation period.

If you're going to stay out of the high risk relapse category, you will need skills to express "current situation" anger in appropriate terms and some tools to get at old, stored anger. Otherwise, minor situations can become major crises. As you immerse yourself in the 12-Step recovery, you'll discover people, books and literature that will offer assistance and insight into resolving past resentments and healing old memories. My chapters, "Emotions Don't Demand Actions" and "Reading Your Richter Scale", might also give you some tips and tools on changing your relationship with anger.

Becoming too lonely usually reflects an isolation pattern. Many times it's easier to be alone than to be with others who are consciously or unconsciously applying pressure on us to be "good" and stick to our commitments concerning food and eating. Isolation is a "hey day" for our disease thinking. If we are left alone inside our heads, just chatting with and listening to the disease voices, we're in trouble. Tell your addiction voices you're "going public"—there will be no more secrets, no more private, internal conversations about eating, food or body image. Find people in recovery that you can regularly interact with and break the isolation pattern. Find people who understand the recovery process and get their help building the supportive recovery voices and exposing the relapse, disease voices. Utilize the O.A. fellowship.

We have usually been living in exhaustion if we've been battling our eating disorder for very long. We've spent money, time and energy looking for a way to fix this baffling problem. The cycle of attempting to control, overcontrol and eventual loss of control is emotionally, mentally and physically tiring. But once we surrender to the fact that the problem is not a moral one, we can give up the battle, the struggle to control. We can be released from exhaustion.

When we do experience feeling tired, it might trigger a flood of old negative feelings that are "memory attached" to the tiredness. The weariness might engulf us in old troublesome feelings. Just recognize them as being old feelings and take some steps to relax. Make a plan to take the edge off the fatigue. Take a few minutes to lie down or soak in a warm tub. Turn on some soft music and find a chair to quietly relax in. Check out your caffeine intake for too much coffee, tea or sodas. Have you been getting the right amount and the right kind of exercise?

Since having an eating disorder doesn't invite balance, most of us won't have a history of balanced living or a sense of how to live a balanced life. We have often lived in extremes—the extremes of going on or off a diet, of over-controlling or loss of all control, eating only healthy foods or eating only junk foods, being on our way up the scale or on our way down the scale, feeling the power of being "perfect" or the self-hate of "failure."

Recovery will demand that we become acquainted with balance. Often in the beginning, we'll mistake it for boredom and it won't feel comfortable. We usually have trouble being without our obsessive focus on our eating problem, on controlling our eating, food or body image. What will we do without these obsessions? . . . with our time and our life?

But take heart, you'll eventually recognize and love serenity. You'll find healthy living invites you to have dreams and goals in a brand new way.

CHAPTER 22
BEING PREPARED FOR SOCIAL OCCASIONS

Most social situations are going to involve eating—weddings, baseball games, backyard bar-b-ques. All major holidays involve the preparation and consuming of food. Getting through these eat-a-thons can be a nightmare when we're first abstaining.

The first option to look at is whether or not this is something you **absolutely** have to do at this time. You might be better off not going with the group to the baseball game right now. Skipping the company pot-luck might be the most comfortable choice in the first 90 days of abstinence. Often we really can postpone an occasion until we've been abstaining a few weeks or months.

If it's a particularly difficult gathering, can you miss it without dire consequences? If you were physically ill and home in bed, would it go on without you? Be honest, make the decision based on your recovery. We don't have to continually avoid social events, but in the beginning it's probably a healthy idea to stay away from the unusually troublesome situations.

When you're certain that attending a function is the best action for you, then make your plan. In your mind, walk through what might happen. Get some feedback. Make an alternate plan. Plans aren't results. Let go of controlling the results. Let go of *others* behavior.

If it's a cocktail party, skip the first hour. Let the hors d'oeuvre "feeding frenzy" die down before arriving. Give yourself permission to leave early if necessary. It's OK *not* to be comfortable and serene in your first few outings.

Making some firm decisions in advance can really quiet the obsessive chattering in our heads. If we are still in the "should I or shouldn't I" or the "will I or won't I" loop, obsession reigns!

Decide, for just this one occasion, to not randomly eat. "We can do for one day what it would appall us to do for a lifetime."

Once we've made the decision to go and be abstinent, some detailed plans might include:

- Take a companion who's committed to the concept of recovery, yours or theirs.
- Plan to call someone after the event to let them know how it went.
- When offered food at a non-meal time, a reply of "No thanks, not right now," usually works great.
- When asked if you tasted or tried a particular dish, a re-sponse of "No, but it looks great. The host always does such a beautiful job," will keep the conversation going and get off the subject of whether or not you're having any.
- When the hostess has done an exceptional job of preparing a dessert to go with coffee later, a reply of "I'm full right now, but may I take a piece home with me for later? It looks wonderful," can give her the acknowledgement she deserves.
- When we're also making food choices based on health decisions, a statement like, "I'm working with a health professional who has suggested I eliminate foods with additives or preservatives in them," or "Sugar has been affecting my overall health so I'm avoiding it," or "I need to lower my cholesterol so I'm not eating much animal protein," usually forestalls urging from others.

Just remember, nutritional eating isn't synonymous with

abstaining.

Most people will be supportive of our pursuing a higher level of health. *Be careful never to sound condescending*—that will invite defensive responses and more discussion. I also don't recommend using dieting phrases such as, "I can't eat that" or "I shouldn't have any" or "I'm trying to lose weight." These phrases will kick in our dieting mentality and lead to interaction we had hoped to avoid.

We're never obligated to answer rude or personal questions. We never need to defend ourselves. My experience was that when I became comfortable with no random eating, others rarely noticed.

Every now and then, a well-meaning friend would begin to discuss my recovery with others. Although the intention was loving, it sometimes caused me embarrassment. I usually smiled and said very little. Sometimes I took the friend aside later and asked them to please not discuss my recovery publicly.

I'm no longer embarrassed to be recovering from an eating disorder and when I have a confident posture, a few sentences like, "I discovered I had an eating disorder and that the way to recover is to not eat in between meals, no matter what," or "The 12 Steps of Alcoholics Anonymous offers a concept that really works on eating disorders too," usually sufficed.

These statements help to eradicate the notion of fat being a moral issue. In addition, they served to increase my self-respect concerning this baffling illness. They may also prove to be a life-preserver to someone else who's secretly suffering from an eating disorder. People's reactions are almost always supportive when *our* understanding and commitment is clear.

Social gatherings are for socializing—enjoy the people and the occasion. If your mind is wrapped up in who's eating what and/or what you're deprived of, you have deprived yourself of the enjoyment of others' company. Think about how you can add to the occasion. Focus on what you can add to life; let go of the focus on self.

Months from now you'll have the experience of knowing you don't have to forego the company of others just because you don't eat in between meals.

CHAPTER 23
KNOW YOUR RELAPSE INDICATORS

In the beginning of recovery from an eating disorder, we can feel lost in a fog of confusion. To lift the fog, we will need to define, separate and clarify the most common obsession issues to become familiar with disease **thinking** before it's disease **behavior.** Staying in the obsessions will keep us relapse prone, so we will want to move through the beginning stage of recovery—move past and free from the obsessions. Part of our recovery will be to recognize and intervene on relapse attitudes and indicators *before* physical relapse occurs.

Obsession issues in recovery from an eating disorder are multifaceted and include three primary obsessions (eating, food and body image) and at least three secondary obsessions (nutrition, exercise and health). Moving past these obsession issues and into living issues will require a thorough understanding of our relapse attitudes and indicators and a level of honesty we didn't bring into recovery with us. It will demand that we challenge our old ideas and define and embrace new ones.

Too many of us never move out of the beginning stage of recovery. We often feel trapped, helplessly focused on these primary and secondary obsessions. Never having the clarity or tools to be free of the obsessions, we never move into the second stage of recovery—into full recovery.

Alcoholics, once they are relieved of the obsession to drink, can begin to deal with living issues. They recognize their part in their problems and understand that the bottles were only a symbol. They begin to recognize the relapse signs that could take them back to drinking—back to choosing between insanity, death or recovery.

Once free of our various obsessions, we who are recovering from eating disorders can also begin to confront our living issues. We can acknowledge that our focus on food and weight was only a symbol. But until we are free of the relentless primary obsessions, any relief from life's issues will seem short lived.

I want to offer some suggestions and insights into how we might be relieved of our multiple obsessions, and to identify some of the most common relapse attitudes and indicators in this beginning phase. Without the fog, we can keep our sights set on recognizing any relapse sign that can take us away from recovery.

To be free of the obsession to **eat**, we must admit to our innermost selves that we have an eating addiction, and over any considerable period we get worse, not better. Letting go of the old idea that *after a considerable period free of the compulsion, we will be normal eaters,* **must** be replaced with the belief that we have a progressive, debilitating and incurable disease that can be arrested, never cured. Understanding and accepting that we have an illness can offer us relief—relief from the insanity of believing that **this** time random eating, or dieting and/or overeating will lead to different results, and relief from the shame of feeling defective and different from others.

For us to experience freedom from the eating obsession, **continuous abstinence will be the key,** abstinence from random eating in between meals and/or randomly including "add ons" that change a meal into a binge. Random eating can ignite the feeding frenzy energy. When we no longer have the option of random eating (when we abstain), we can be free of the obsession to eat. The thoughts about eating in between meals might come and go, but when we no longer take them seriously, when we no longer act on them, they are simply disease thoughts, not obsession.

The obsession with **food** is as cunning, baffling and powerful as the obsession to eat. First we're told to abstain from addictive eating no matter what, and then we're told that to recover we must change our relationship with food and body. It feels like an impossible task.

Just take it piecemeal, one day at a time, one meal at a time, one awareness at a time, one new belief at a time. We can live the adage, "a journey of a thousand miles begins with the first step."

In the beginning, for a comfortable abstinence, we might want to avoid our favorite binge foods. If a certain food seems to set up a craving, leave it alone for awhile and don't reintroduce it without planning and support. **But if it sets up a craving when you avoid it, plan a moderate serving of it into your menu with support and openness.** Be willing to check your motives at "gut level" when doing your menu planning. Be willing to answer this question honestly, "Does this food choice feed the disease or does it feed the recovery?" Don't settle for an impulsive relation-ship with your favorite binge foods.

When I first started abstaining, I avoided my favorite binge foods—french fries and chocolate chip cookies—for a while. After arriving at a moderate, stable weight, I reintroduced both of my favorite binge foods, one at a time, with a plan and much support. French fries came first. I ate them in a restaurant, accompanied by a supportive person. I ate them in a moderate portion with a moderate meal. It seemed to take all the power and craving away from french fries. Today, I might eat french fries five or six times a year, always in a restaurant. I never cook them at home.

Chocolate chip cookies came after the french fries experiment. I planned a meal with two cookies as the dessert. I had successfully eaten other desserts, always in moderation. I had discovered that one of the justifications I used for the late-night, half-the-cake snack, was deprivation and restriction. A small piece of dessert included with my dinner took the power and craving away from dessert foods. *I had realized that the disease always wanted to continue eating and eating.* I'd reinforce my new belief by repeating, **I have the disease, but I'm not the disease.** Still, planning a meal that included two chocolate chip cookies felt very risky. Everything went fine, I had a little craving and some uncomfortable feelings. **But I realized that there was no food craving that could justify breaking my abstinence.** Today, I might eat chocolate chip cookies once or twice a month. I don't feel deprived, but then I'm willing to go to any lengths to have a **comfortable** abstinence.

Before we tackle body image issues (that's the next chapter), I want to suggest some writings you can do to help you clarify and surrender the eating and food obsessions.

1. Write a definition of abstinence, one you can live with 100 percent of the time, one that reflects 100 percent surrender, one that offers continuous recovery. (one that arrests all the addictive eating behaviors)
2. Write a definition of healthy eating, one you can live with 60-75 percent of the time.
3. Write a definition of healthy nourishing—physically, emotionally, mentally, and spiritually.
4. List the characteristics of a healthy relationship with eating, food and body.

Next, write a history of your eating/weight problem. Pay close attention to all the ways and how many times you set yourself up to return to an active eating/weight problem. You'll probably notice that emotional relapse **thinking** usually came before emotional relapse **behavior**. *Both dieting thinking and dieting actions feed the obsessions and the eventual return to disease living.* As you record your eating problem history, you will start to recognize the dieting mentality, with all its subtleties and dangerous pitfalls.

To be adequately prepared to challenge the old ways, and ideas and to substitute new beliefs, attitudes and behaviors, you'll need to make a master list of *your* most common relapse indicators/attitudes. Although we all have our own individual ones, the following are some of the most common relapse attitudes and behaviors.

- always eating alone
- never eating alone
- "this won't be enough" mentality
- calorie counting
- baking for others
- gourmet cooking
- allowing "add ons" after starting to eat
- keeping secrets with food
- keeping secrets with laxatives
- keeping secrets with exercising
- wearing clothes too big and/or loose
- wearing clothes too small and/or tight
- excessive focus on nutrition
- excessive focus on a food plan
- excessive focus on health issues
- knowing what and where all the food in the house is
- "as soon as I'm at my goal weight, I'll be OK" mentality
- choosing foods/liquids based on calories, not nutritional value
- constantly **thinking** about what we're going to eat/not eat to be OK
- constantly **talking** about what we're going to eat/not eat to be OK
- staying filled up with liquids
- buying or cooking large quantities
- "this little extra won't matter" mentality

- staring into the refrigerator
- excessive gum chewing
- "if only my thighs were smaller, I'd be OK" mentality
- "if only I were 15 lbs. thinner, I'd be OK" mentality

Next, make an intervention plan, a plan to interrupt thinking and actions that feed the obsessions. For example, plan an action that takes you away from a "slippery" situation, an inaction that keeps you in a safe environment when you feel driven to act on compulsive/impulsive energy, a question to challenge an old idea, an affirmation to strengthen a new idea. Some additional suggestions to include in your relapse prevention plan are:

- leaving the kitchen (or where ever) for a two minute break
- telling yourself, "it's only a meal"
- reminding yourself, "nothing tastes as good as abstinence/ recovery feels"
- asking, "Do I have the energy to live in the disease, **again?**"
- repeating, "eat to nourish, not control"
- calling a friend in recovery
- reading over your eating/dieting history
- asking, "Does this feed the disease, or does it feed the recovery?"
- reading a chapter out of this book
- repeating out loud, to someone in recovery, anything your internal, disease chattering voices say to you about eating, food or body
- reading anything out of the **Overeaters Anonymous** book
- attending an O.A. meeting
- repeating a recovery slogan, over and over
- reminding yourself, "looks are just for looking at"
- repeating, "One meal at a time, one day at a time"

- planning social eating events in advance, having a backup plan, and then letting go of the actual results

With your relapse prevention plan in hand, read the next chapter and include information on the #1 relapse problem, body image. I invite you to believe you never have to go into physical relapse again.

CHAPTER 24

BODY IMAGE: #1 RELAPSE PROBLEM

Body image is probably the number one relapse problem in the beginning of recovery. Just as a child with asthma might learn to manipulate others with his asthma attacks and unconsciously begin to define himself as being defective, many of us also unconsciously define ourselves as defective and develop a style of manipulating our environment through our relationship with our body/body image—through our disease.

For us to attempt to make a searching and fearless inventory of our body image beliefs, we must first be committed to continuous abstinence and, secondly, to not manipulating or "playing" with our food, meals or **quantity**. The following questions will help you conclude whether you're ready to address your body image obsession.

1. Are you willing to go to any length to stay abstinent?
2. Are you willing to go to any length to have a **comfortable** abstinence?
3. Are you willing to go to any length to recover?
4. Are you willing to believe that there is a power greater than yourself?
5. Are you willing to believe that a Higher Power can supply all the power you need to abstain?
6. Do you believe it's in your highest and best interest to stay abstinent 100 percent of the time?
7. Do you believe it's in your highest and best interest to have a healthy relationship with food, eating and your body?
8. Are you willing to believe that the body nature intended you to have will "show up" if you abstain and work the 12-Steps?
9. Do you have a Higher Power you can trust?

If you can honestly answer yes to the preceding questions, then you're ready to look closely at your body image issues. If you can't answer yes to all of the questions, take the time to explore the questions you answered no to. Get out the paper and pen. Find out what stands in the way of you responding affirmatively.

Overweight, underweight or "goal" weight, we have a vague feeling that body size and shape is not the answer to our safety and serenity. But lacking an awareness of how we've misused our focus on weight and body image, we will continue to pretend a certain body size and shape can and will give us all that we've yearned for.

I've noticed there are three common issues that surface when we begin to deal with body image. Although we all might have an understanding of these different issues, for some of us the accompanying delusions have become major blocks to our continuous recovery and peace of mind.

1. Sexuality Issues—the delusion that a certain weight can and will set a safe sexual boundary for us.

    •   when we don't know how to say no, and/or we don't know how to say yes, we pretend our weight or body size will keep the questions away.
    •   when we don't understand why we don't have loving, intimate relationships, we pretend our body size and shape is why.
    •   when we don't know how to evaluate the love of others, we test them with our weight, or weight gain, and pretend that if they stay with us no matter what our body size, then they really do love us.

2. Power/Safety Issues—the delusion that a certain weight will set a safe physical boundary for us.

- when a five-pound weight loss feels like 50 and fear sets in, we pretend our body size can physically protect us from others and we regain the lost pounds.

- when we approach a "goal" weight and feel we're shrinking in height and stature, fear will tell us we're losing our power and control in life, so we pretend our body size, with our 15 - 25 pound buffer, is the magic to stabilizing power and control.

- when we start to shed our weight, fear tells us that it's coming off too quickly and our health is in jeopardy, so we pretend that regaining the pounds will make us healthy again.

- when a five-pound weight gain reflects an adult body in the mirror, we pretend a child's body will protect us from adult responsibilities and we begin the starving and/or binge purge cycle again.

3. Grief Issues—the delusion that obsessive focus on weight and body size will set a safe emotional boundary for us.

    - when we experience the loss of our childhood or childhood dreams, disappointment and pain tells us it's safer to focus on achieving a "goal" weight, so we pretend that a "perfect" body will reflect a "perfect" history.

    - when we experience the loss of a loved one, pain and denial tell us it's easier to focus on achieving the "right" body than to re-feel those past memories, so we live in the silence of "time will take care of it."

    - when we experience the loss of a God that we can trust to protect us, terror tells us not to look back, so we pretend that attempting to control our body size and shape will keep us alive and safe. Sometimes the terror is so great and the controlling so exhausting, we prefer to die, using our disease as the vehicle.

Set aside time to write down your emotional reactions to these ten different concepts. Search your history for these patterns or similar ones. It will help to get a very clear picture of **how** you've used your disease to protect you from feelings and memories, **how** you've used your disease to set survival boundaries and **how** you've used it to deal with life.

When we finally commit to letting go of using our disease to interact with life, we almost always will be bombarded with "codependency" issues—living issues. Codependency is when we unhappily and sometimes unconsciously *live from our history,* not from our own adult, mature self. Boundary setting problems are always codependency issues. If there is one point, in addition to eating disorders being a disease, I would want you to hear, it is this: For continuous, quality recovery, **you must address and resolve your codependency issues.**

There are many good books that give insight and direction to codependency recovery. There is also a 12-Step group called Codependents Anonymous. Seek them out as soon as possible.

Now, another powerful piece of information, *the idea that looks are just for looking at.* **Wow, what a concept!** To believe that we're not our looks, that we're not loved for our looks and that physical appearance is not the best criteria to use when choosing friends and/or lovers might be heresy in this culture, but for us it will be an absolute necessity to move this important concept from our head to our heart. It can create an attitude of happy, joyous and free.

The *looks are just for looking at* concept has, for many years, been my quick and easy challenge when the old beliefs and ideas about the importance of "looks" begin to surface. As an affirmation, it has been a valuable link to reinforcing the new beliefs. When phrased as the question, "Do I want to be involved with someone who values me just for my body or looks?" it helps me to pull honesty back into my thinking.

Once we are armed with the exact nature of how in the past we used the obsessive focus on our body size and shape, we might begin to notice that the mirrors in our lives cease being "fun house" mirrors. You know those mirrors that can reflect a 20-pound weight change in the blink of an eye? The fun house mirror phenomenon will begin to disappear.

As our clarity about body image issues sharpens and our acceptance of the disease concept deepens, the self-hate that often manifested itself in the mirror will begin to dissipate.

Our body image attitudes will either be the final door to freedom or a revolving door to obsession and relapse.

CHAPTER 25
INNER FAMILY HEALING

In this chapter, I want to share with you some of my concepts about how codependency and eating disorder issues can become enmeshed during our childhood, and how that enmeshment can stunt our recovery from our eating disorder.

When we've used our eating disorder to adapt in a dysfunctional environment, our eating disorder gets intertwined with our codependency issues. If we have used our eating disorder compulsion and obsessions for protection, to set boundaries and/or to avoid feelings, beginning physical recovery from our eating disorder can trigger free-floating fear and terror and/or grief and loss. We will experience the loss of the "tool" that we have unconsciously viewed as beneficial—our eating disorder!

When this happens, instead of abstinence offering us more and more emotional and spiritual serenity, acquiring an average size body and/or being relieved of our obsessions can create more and more turmoil and confusion. We don't fully understand why we begin to "play" with our food quantity and quality, again, why we put weight back on or why, with all our knowledge about our disease and the recovery, we are seduced back into obsessive thinking, emotional relapse and sometimes physical relapse.

"Inner family" work can begin to separate our codependency issues from our eating disorder issues. It can make recovery clearer and simpler. When you know "who" it is that used the extra weight for protection, you can begin to listen to that historical, younger self share the feelings and experiences that led to the dire need for physical and/or sexual safety. When you know which past self it was that felt safer obsessively focusing on food or body image rather than acknowledging the trauma or chaos around them, you can begin to discuss with them the memories and experiences that helped create a "solution" that has now become a major block to full recovery.

There are many books and workshops now available that offer valuable information about our inner child, how to become acquainted with that wonderful child and how to heal past experiences, memories and feelings. They help guide us to healthy self-parenting.

I suggest beginning some visualization work that includes **various past selves,** not just the magical and wounded inner child. Find the essence (and maybe a few photos) of yourself—of several younger "yous," usually as a very young child (under three), maybe a middle-age child (six to eleven), and always include at least one teenager (twelve to 18). Sometimes a pre-puberty child and middle teen will both have powerful information for you. If you're 30 years old, you probably have a couple of past selves in their twenties that hold memories and experiences that need re-evaluating and reintegrating. And if you're 50 years old . . . well, you get the idea.

Depending on your individual history, amend and alter my visualization ideas to fit your needs.

A beginning visualization that often sets the stage for getting acquainted with "who is it that needs to talk," is to create a safe setting in your mind's eye. Visualize a room with warm lighting and comfortable things to sit on. Place yourself in the center of a circle and invite your inner family members in to make up the surrounding circle. The goals of this beginning visualization are:

- acknowledgement and awareness of the different selves as your inner family

- to communicate your willingness to take the lead in learning new ways to set safe emotional, intellectual, physical and sexual boundaries
- to express your commitment to love and care for them in healthy ways

As you use this beginning meditation over and over, always try to communicate the essence of these points. After regular "meetings" with your newly found inner family, the visualization usually takes on a very creative element. Your inner family will start to initiate communication with you. The inner selves begin to trust your commitment to them. They are aware of your recovery footwork and they've gotten to know and bond with each other.

One of them might tell you how they used the compulsion and the extra weight to avoid feeling small and unprotected. Another self might tell you how they obsessively focused on food and body image to avoid experiencing feelings of failure and disappointment. These inner selves hold valuable information that can be the key to inner healing, a powerful healing.

I encourage you to honor their feelings and experiences by just listening, not judging or shaming. Tell them about O.A. and Co.D.A.'s 12-Step recovery programs. Tell them about your new Higher Power, *about the God of your understanding*. Gently invite them to believe it's possible to let go of all the eating disorder obsessions, that it's OK to trust a Higher Power and you to keep them safe. Tell them about your commitment to live by the spiritual principles expressed in the 12 Steps. Ask them to join you in your recovery journey.

Our eating disorder will tell us to eat over anything, everything and nothing, so a decision to abstain from compulsive overeating, no matter what, will be absolutely necessary while traveling this

path. If we are to begin to listen to the small inner voices that know the old ways and old beliefs bring more pain than comfort, we must stop shoving food down their throats to quiet them, we must not starve them to experience feelings of power, and we must not repeat the shaming and rejecting that they've experienced in the past.

There is a way to stop the inner turmoil—abstain a day at a time, no matter what, and seek the tools to live the spiritual principles at an inner level as well as an outer level.

CHAPTER 26
FIND, DEVELOP AND USE A SUPPORT SYSTEM

Overeaters Anonymous can be a lifeline of support in recovery, but if you don't live in an area where there are meetings, or the meetings in your area are full of the dieting mentality, here are some tips on ways to build a support system.

Seek a professional who understands alcoholism and the 12-Step recovery process and ask them to be part of your support system. If you already have a therapist, doctor, chiropractor, etc., ask them to read this book and support your commitment to recovery.

If you're active in a church group, share this book with them and ask them to support your understanding of the illness and your spiritual commitment to recovery.

Attend some open Alcoholics Anonymous meetings and listen to members share their recovery. Listen to how hopeless and defeated they felt and how, now, they have a solution. If you're approached about why you're attending A.A. meetings, a simple response that you have discovered you have an eating disorder, that it's an addictive disease like alcoholism and you're trying to understand how to use the 12 Steps of recovery to arrest your illness, will usually be an adequate answer.

Write to O.A. World Service, P.O. Box 44020, Rio Rancho, NM 87174-4020 and ask for a "pen pal" in recovery and/or the phone numbers of the closest members in your state. Utilize the recovering community in your state. Request information on how you can order the book, Overeaters Anonymous. Purchase it and read it. Ask for a contact in a city where you are planning to vacation; write in advance and plan on attending some meetings when you travel.

If you have a best friend who knows your struggle, ask him or her to read this book with you. Create a plan that will offer you understanding and support for your change.

Sometimes our families have been negatively affected by this disease and they will need a little time before they can be a good resource. Often they are as caught up in the dieting mentality as we are. And sometimes their behavior will look and feel like sabotage, because of the fear triggered in them when you begin to change, and you are no longer the sick one, the weak one or the fat one.

If you do have O.A. meetings in your area but you find them dominated by the dieting/weight control mentality, or with little or no commitment to continuous abstinence, it usually means they don't yet have an understanding of eating disorders as an addictive disease. The chapter in the O.A. book entitled, "Our Invitation to You," will shed all the light you need to start your 12-Step recovery. Read it and share it, over and over. See if it's possible to recruit others onto your support team.

There's an old saying, "When we finally get teachable, the teacher shows up." Well, when we get supportable, the supporters will show up. A favorite saying that I made up in the beginning of my recovery is, "God will send me whomever I need, when I need them, for whatever I need them for, for however long I need them." It brought me great comfort and it was sure a faith-building affirmation. If I kept my eyes open and didn't gripe about which face and name the teacher/supporter came attached to, it worked wonderfully.

CHAPTER 27
LOOKING FOR "GRANDMAS"

Part of your support team might be people I like to call "Grandmas." Grandmas can be older than you or younger than you. They can be of the same sex or the opposite sex. They might be relatives, they might be friends.

A Grandma is someone who honors you as a person. Someone who celebrates your essence. They are constantly reflecting back to you your unique talents and inner beauty. A Grandma will subtly, and sometimes not so subtly, invite you to be all you can be. They will rejoice in supporting your dreams. They will offer comfort during a seeming failure and they will stick by you in your successes.

We will need to continue to parent, or re-parent, ourselves. Grandmas won't fight your battles or fix you or your life. They will use love to invite you to grow and they will use appropriate, loving honesty. A Grandma is someone who's in your corner, no matter what.

They're not saints or gods. A Grandma won't be able to be all of those things every moment and they might not always be available every time you need them, but they will **always be on your team**—never in an adversary role.

Very few people really understand how to **be** a Grandma and few of us, when in our codependency fog, will be able to recognize them or their value to us. But it's a certainty that having a couple of Grandmas in our lives can make a miraculous difference in the way we feel about ourselves and the way we choose to live.

Some of us have never had one, but many of us have experienced the Grandma phenomenon in a real grandparent. Maybe our only interaction with a Grandma was a neighbor who loved and adored us or perhaps a teacher who saw something special in us that others seemed unable to acknowledge.

The change that our recovery invites, or demands, will sometimes meet resistance in our immediate environment. When we've been part of the delicate balance that contributes to a dysfunctional environment, our changes will instinctively be seen as a threat to the emotional safety of others and sometimes as a threat of abandonment—abandonment of them and the old way of living.

Don't be surprised if things seem to get worse before they get better. But in the mean time, keep your eyes open for Grandmas. A Grandma could be a most valuable asset in the uncertainty and fear that change can create. When you spot one, be willing to take the time to nourish and nurture the friendship.

Chapter 28
REMEMBER YOUR LAST DIET &/OR BINGE

We have this interesting little quirk in our thinking. After a day, week or month of freedom from our food and eating obsession, we say, "Well, that's finally over with!" After a period of normalcy, we assume we're normal and that the eating or weight problem is a thing of the past.

We don't go through this cycle once, we go through it many times. Selective recall is a common problem in all addictive diseases. The thought that, "This time it will be different," is common to alcoholics when they take that first drink and to compulsive overeaters when we take that random bite, when we plan that first binge or when we justify that **larger than large** meal.

We have the automatic ability to deny our track record. We refuse to remember the humiliation of a weight gain, the self-hate triggered by being overweight. We refuse to recall the deprivation we endured when starving or dieting, the stress of trying to be in constant control. We refuse to remember the self-loathing of vomiting. And, we refuse to connect the power-rush of dieting and exercising as a set up for the loss of control cycle.

We will need to eliminate selective recall if we want to be free. A great suggestion is to write out your weight and eating history. Go as far back as you can remember, don't get into blame or minimizing, just take an observational fact-finding tour. We usually have some early childhood memories about an *odd* relationship with food or eating. Usually some powerful feelings about our bodies and food during adolescence. And most of us, during adulthood, have a history of various attempts to control—diets, starving, over-the-counter diet pills, excessive exercising and sometimes, illegal diet pills, vomiting and laxative abuse. Highlight every attempt to control and how long each lasted. Read it once a week for a month or so.

Write out one of your last diets. What it felt like to have to start again, what it felt like going through it and **off it**. Read it over once a day for a few weeks and whenever you recognize selective recall popping up.

Write out one of your last binges. Detail all the actions and feelings, especially the ones at the end. How did your binge end? What did it feel like the next morning? Read it once a day along with the accounting of your last diet.

I suggest you never throw these valuable records away. They'll keep your memory green and promote honesty and reality. One of our best defenses against a relapse is remembering our history and **knowing** we have an addictive disease.

Chapter 29
EMOTIONS DON'T DEMAND ACTIONS

Our feelings and our relationship to our feelings have probably been the topic of endless conversations—internally and/or externally. We judge them, act on them inappropriately, convert them into ones we think are more acceptable, and sometimes feel totally run by them and/or completely shut off from them. But typically, emotions aren't random. They're connected to our perceptions, attitudes and beliefs. Their roots are in our personal history and in our relationship to that history.

A primitive Indian who interprets thunder as God's wrath will emote and act differently than a modern day meteorologist. If he believes that God punishes, and specifically punishes him, hearing the thunder can bring fear, terror and the act of escaping or hiding—an entirely different emotional reaction to thunder than that of our present day scientist!

As we start our 12-Step recovery process, we are immediately asked to take in the belief that eating disorders are an illness, a disease that, like alcoholism, is an addictive disease. When we take on this new idea, we usually haven't completely let go of the old moral issue idea.

During that beginning stage, as we consciously and deliberately act as if we believe the new idea and not the old, we might experience the emotional confusion of holding two conflicting ideas simultaneously. Emotions will sometimes flow from the dieting mentality and sometimes flow from the recovering mentality.

As we immerse ourselves in a community or support system that is also approaching eating disorder recovery from an addictive disease position, surrender and acceptance becomes more and more a spontaneous reaction, both emotionally and physically.

An addiction will talk to us in sentences—ones that reflect "yearning for" and "planning to get" dialogue. When we begin to identify these voices as belonging to the disease, not to the recovery—**not to us**— we begin to respond with different emotions. Instead of the old response to the unexplainable driving need to eat, we might respond with, "Oh yeah, that's just disease chatter. I have an eating disorder *but* I'm not the eating disorder."

Instead of the old yearning=planning=doing=remorse cycle, we can say to ourself, "Sure I want to eat (manipulate food or weight), I have an eating disorder. I just don't have to act on the feelings." We no longer have to be afraid of the thoughts and feelings, we've made a decision to **act on** our new attitude, our new ideas.

Just because we **want** to eat, binge, snack, graze or skip a meal, it doesn't mean we have to do it. Most us have wanted to quit our job and even thought seriously about it, but the thoughts and feelings don't demand action. Some of us have even wanted to break the law at one time or another, but decided that the consequences out-weighed the feeling. I want to invite you to believe that wanting to randomly eat, skip a meal and/or overeat doesn't mean you have to.

When we've lived for years acting on those disease thoughts and feelings, it will be an enormous task to surrender and accept the new ideas, new directions and new actions. As we change our relationship with our past, and as we change our relationship with our present, we will notice feelings and emotions change. They will be flowing from the new beliefs.

Recovery will include the process of becoming aware of a full range of emotions. Working O.A.'s Steps will demand an insightful searching of our past situations, perceptions, reactions and emotions. Living the spiritual principles reflected in the Steps will involve an ongoing experience of being fully human—**and the state of perfection in humans is imperfection!**

CHAPTER 30
READING YOUR RICHTER SCALE

Over the years, I've used writing as a tool for self-discovery—for dialoguing with my inner selves, dialoguing with my God, and for identifying old ideas and integrating new ones. In this chapter, I want to share with you my style of writing that addresses the latter. I'll go through it step by step in the hope that you, too, might find it a beneficial tool.

1. I sit down to write when my emotional reaction doesn't equal the situation, when my "Richter Scale" hits 9.5 and an appropriate reaction is 2.0. For example, my car breaks down on the freeway making me late for an appointment; if I want to call Suicide Prevention, not the auto club, I know it's time to write!

2. I begin by asking myself questions, "What am I feeling?" "Why am I so upset?" I attempt to answer by describing the feelings in as much detail as possible, i.e., "I'm so sad that I could sit and cry for three days" or "I'm so angry I want to sue the car mechanic." This exaggerated, detailed description aids me in discovering the exact feeling and intensity.

3. Then I guess at what might be triggering such an intense emotional response. I just start making up explanations that would make sense based on my history, such as, "Could it be that by being late to my appointment, I think 'their' opinion of me will be lowered and I will lose esteem in their eyes?" or "Could it be that by being late, I will disappoint my colleagues (or friends), and they'll think I don't care enough about them to be on time?" Or maybe, "Could it be that I want to blame the car mechanic for my car trouble, for my

missed appointment and for the fact that I will owe others an explanation and an apology?" or "Could it be that feeling blame is easier than feeling shame?" or "Could it be that my self-worth is contingent on being prompt?"

4. My body will tell me when I hit on my answer. I call it a **recognition response.** My physical and emotional bodies both react. I might cry or get teary when I recognize my answer. I might feel that "ah ha" awareness when the information strikes a cord in my heart.

5. Then I explore the hidden beliefs behind the emotional and physical reactions. I start the next sentence with, "I'm acting as if I believe . . ." I continue to write until the underlying, old, negative, spiritual ideas surface. For example, "I'm acting as if my whole career hinges on this one appointment" or "I'm acting as if being late one time will erase my colleagues positive opinion of me." Or maybe, "I'm acting as if I won't be able to find the appropriate words to respectfully explain my lateness" or "I'm acting as if car problems are more powerful than God's influence in my life."

6. I finish my writing by affirming a new spiritual belief. Such as, "Even when I don't like or approve of what's happening in my life, I will accept it and look for the lessons to be learned" or "I no longer need to allow outside situations to be the sole deciding factor for my state of mind" or "Today I know God's timing is perfect in every area of my life even if I cannot see it" or "No harm can come to me unless it's for my highest good."

If we're going to let go of all our old ideas, we'll need new ones to replace them. You might want to make a list of your old ideas and make a list of the ideals you would prefer to live. Answer the question, "What would a healthy person think about and do for self and others?" Develop a sane and sound ideal of the person that you and your Higher Power would want you to be. Check it out with someone you admire, maybe someone who has a functional, peaceful way of life. It was one of my goals in recovery to become a woman I respect—the woman God would have me be!

CHAPTER 31
IS THERE LIFE AFTER ABSTINENCE?

Answering this question is, consciously or unconsciously, one of our biggest concerns. ***We dread living with our disease and we dread living without it.*** As much as we've hoped and prayed to live as normal eaters, living in recovery—living without an active disease—is often experienced as a loss. The loss of the driving compulsion and obsessions sometimes makes us feel like we've lost a reason to live. We've often spent years in this destructive relationship and now that we're free of it, the void feels like the loss of an old friend. Yes, we've had our difficulties in this relationship, but it was oddly comfortable to be caught up in an ongoing struggle. "At least I knew what to expect," we say. Now we wonder how to deal with this "new" life.

When the beginning stage of recovery offers us a life free of struggle, we may question whether this *freedom from* can or will offer us *freedom to*.

This new found freedom usually leaves us with the realization that we're left with our past—past feelings and experiences. Most of us will need, and want, a thorough healing of our victim memories but for a truly thorough healing, *we will need to include a responsible awareness of our part in any victimizing and/or abusive actions or roles toward others.* My first sense of being truly human came from finding enough forgiveness and acceptance to surround **both** experiences.

If we've surrendered to the reality that we have a disease, have worked the 12 Steps on all our eating disorder obsessions and have begun to explore how we've used our disease to deal with life, we have arrived at the second stage of recovery. We are now somewhat prepared to face life on life's terms.

As we move into this second stage of recovery where we no longer use or need our disease, we may begin to experience some new fears—fear of success, fear of being average, fear of letting go of the old excuses we used to justify not pursuing goals and dreams.

In the middle stage of recovery, our codependency recovery tools and insights prove to be the healing force that moves us forward. We begin to discover what **we** really like and what unique talents we possess. We begin to acquire healthy passions for living, sometimes for the first time.

When all of our "head" information moves that most important 18 inches down to our heart, we begin to feel like a channel for creativity instead of a receptacle for engulfing feelings and pain.

We begin to possess the right and the ability to dream, achieve, fail and succeed. I found the right to simply **BE.** As long as I honored myself and others by living from spiritual principles, I found I can remain a woman I admire and respect. I found real inner peace.

As I started to transform dreams into goals, **I came to believe that spiritually, there is no real competition, no real rejection, no real success and no real failure, only me being guided down a divine path.** Now, rejection and failure are simply words I use to describe the need to try a different path—a different direction. Success is a word I use to describe the experience of being the channel for my Higher Power.

I began to believe the universe just uses these situations to guide and direct me to where I need to be. Even with all of its curves, risks and limited view, traveling down destiny's road brought a magical discovery. I discovered that acceptance of today brings serenity and joy, acceptance of the past brings forgiveness and understanding and that acceptance of the future brings freedom and faith.

Is there life after abstinence? My answer is "Yes, and hang on tight 'cause you're in for an incredible journey!!"

PART II

FROM THE AUTHOR

Becky Lu Jackson

My story is not about finding the villains or events that gave me an eating problem. Although I do believe that environmental influences are a key ingredient in the unfoldment of this complex disorder, I also believe that, in addition to environmental factors, there is a biological predisposition at the root of this illness. **But** its driving energy is based in how we personally reacted to life **and** to having the illness.

I now see how I unconsciously used my dysfunctional eating to survive my younger years and how I had to let go of it to survive my adult years. As odd as it might sound, at times I have felt lucky to have had compulsive eating available to that younger Becky.

Many of the details of my early history are recounted from my mother's memories and many I recalled as an adult looking back over my life. As I describe the memories of my childhood, adolescence and young adulthood—as I share my recollections of past events, experiences and perceptions—my purpose is to acquaint you with me, the author. To share my history, my struggle and my recovery. My recovery from compulsive overeating, diet pill induced starving and alcoholic drinking.

I had an awareness of "something wrong" with my eating since I was a small child. For years my mom told a story about me as a baby. She always told it in a humorous way, none of us realizing it was a reflection of my odd relationship with food. She said that when I was still crawling, probably about ten months old, I "ran" away from home. The story goes that we lived a couple of houses away from the corner ice cream parlor and I crawled down there and said "vanilla." This is probably not an accurate version but an embellished one. Nevertheless, it was more than likely based on some truth about my driving interest in food and eating.

I was a thin, active middle-age child. Sometimes I would overeat to the point of spontaneously vomiting; other times I'd have no interest in eating at all. I didn't understand that driving need to eat. All I knew was when it hit, I felt powerless over it.

I remember the driving need to continue eating often kicked in at dinner. At the end of dinner, I'd ask my mom what was left over. I'd tell her I was still hungry and she would always let me eat whatever food was left. If it was lima beans, I'd finish them off; if it was fried chicken, I'd finish it off; if it was liver and onions, I would eat all that was left. At times I would eat so much I'd get "sick" and vomit; I always assumed the food itself made me sick—not the *quantity* of food. For years I avoided chicken and lima beans because I thought *they* were the problem. No one seemed aware of my periodic, out-of-control eating. There didn't seem to be any consequences; I wasn't fat.

As a young adult, I did the same thing with my drinking—if I experienced a physical reaction to over-drinking, I'd switch substances—I'd switch from gin to vodka, from vodka to wine. For years I assumed it was a particular liquor or wine, not the *quantity* that caused the reactions.

Historically, I was born just at the end of World War II. My father, after eight years of marriage, asked for a divorce while my mother was pregnant with me. My mother, who was a housewife caring for my two-year-old sister, desperately wanted the family to stay together but my father had gotten involved with another woman and wanted a divorce so that he could marry her. Although the divorce provided my mother with property and enough income so she didn't need to work, it also brought her great sadness and grief.

When I was about one year old, my mother decided to take her two daughters and move from Texas to Colorado, away from the heartache of watching the man she loved build a new life with a new family. When she informed my father about her plans to move away, he reacted with feelings of loss and upset. He devised a plan to "bring her to her senses." He decided to not return us at the end of visitation day. Instead he called her from an undisclosed location and begged her to reconsider the decision to move.

Many of the details are no longer clear but within about a week he did return us to my mom and she continued with the plans to move. Only much later in life did I realize how traumatizing that one week away from my mother was. My reaction to the prolonged, engulfing terror of being motherless seemed to set up a pattern of almost complete repression of fear.

By the time I was about two years old, we had resettled in Colorado. My mom remarried when I was about three and my stepfather seemed to me like the world's greatest dad. The thing that made him great was I felt loved and adored by him. When I looked at him, his eyes seemed to reflect unconditional acceptance and love.

My sister and I continued to visit my birth-father yearly but I don't recall knowing him in a personal, intimate way. I only saw him and his new family from an observational position for many years. Later on I discovered that my mother's drinking may have played an important part in my birth-father's decision to divorce her.

When I was ten years old, I recall my mom asking me if her drinking bothered me. I told her I'd like it better if she didn't drink. We had the conversation when she wasn't drinking and she responded sympathetically. I was startled the next time I saw her drinking and said, "I thought you said you wouldn't drink anymore?" She responded by saying "No, I didn't say I'd stop, I just asked you how you felt about it."

I was stunned and hurt. However, only through retrospection in sobriety would I recognize how deeply hurt I was and how I used my teenage drinking as a retaliation to return the hurt.

In my grade school years I had an out-going, optimistic style. I was well liked at school—the most popular boy in class had a crush on me. I was bright, pretty and in the gifted group. Scholastic achievement was relatively easy for me. I took dancing and acrobatics; I dearly loved the time I spent in those classes.

My mother was a WASP, (White, Anglo-Saxon, Protestant) from the South. She thought of us as "better than." She was preoccupied with "ranking" others—who was better than who. With my friends, in the neighborhood or at school, I too, constantly compared myself with others. I could almost always adjust my perspective to see myself as better-than. This attitude was impossible to hide from others, but surprisingly, I remained popular at school up until junior high. Sadly, I might add, my older sister often received the brunt of my subtle, hurtful comparisons.

My mother, step-dad and teachers seemed to reinforce my arrogance and precocious independence. To the outside world I appeared super-mature and in-control for the first 12 years of my life.

During the last few weeks of elementary school, the tide turned. My girl friends finally rebelled against my tyranny. As a group, they confronted me about my controlling, gossiping, obnoxious behavior and "dumped" me, refusing even to talk to me. I was devastated! I began my years at junior high without my supportive entourage of friends, unable to recognize fear and lacking the skills to make the necessary amends or changes to re-establish those grade school relationships.

By the time I completed the seventh grade I had tried alcohol and cigarettes and had found a group of new friends I could feel better-than. I felt somewhat secure again. The first time I drank I blacked out, laughed a lot and thought it was great fun.

I began traveling down a path that caused my mom great pain. Unconsciously, I think I liked the fact that my actions and new friends caused her disappointment and pain. Those were the feelings I experienced as I helplessly watched her abusive drinking, and now she would know what it felt like to watch someone you love harm themselves and others with their drinking. I guess my unconscious thought was, if she wouldn't stop doing what caused me such pain, at least I could cause her some similar pain. I could get even.

As the destructive life-style that goes with teenage drinking accelerated, things at home and school got worse and worse. I was painting myself into a corner with no way out.

By the time I was 15 years old and in the tenth grade, things were unbearable at home. After a series of blow-ups and physical confrontations at home, I secretly packed my bags. One final confrontation brought me to the point of yelling at my mom that my bags were packed and I was prepared to leave. She said the only place she'd let me go was to live with my birth-father.

I called him that night and asked him if I could come and live with him. I gave him no details, the request was just out of the blue, but he said yes anyway. This was my way out of the very destructive life I had built up around myself. I left for Texas, a new family and a new school in the middle of my sophomore year.

In Colorado, my grades had steadily gone down. I had even received a D on my report card. Now, I felt I had an opportunity to start afresh. I began to take high school seriously. I started to study and get good grades again. I knew that if I wanted to get out from under the control of other people, I'd better get a high school diploma.

Settling in Houston, I picked somewhat "safer" people to run around with. In Colorado, I ran around with a rock band and friends who were into drinking and drug selling. Now I picked jazz musicians to focus on and although I continued to drink and do some drug taking, it all seemed much calmer and more mature.

I was still thin and my eating was only periodically out of control. I even enjoyed the out-of-control eating—I would plan what I called "eat-a-thons" with two thin friends who ate the way I did.

My presence in my birth-father's home wreaked havoc. My dad and step-mom made it clear that much of my behavior was unacceptable, but somehow they seemed able to accept *me*. They weren't manipulative. They didn't withhold approval, affection or my allowance.

My stay with them only lasted from February to August. I was asked to move back to my mother's home. My mom had been devastated by my leaving and had been wanting me to come home. I got to return to Colorado on new footing with my mom, with a chance to pick different friends and with a new commitment to my education. I never slowed down on my eating or drinking but I was definitely picking a calmer crowd to do it with.

Back in Denver, I saw how the brief time I spent with my birth-father and his family had given me new information about family life. I intuitively knew they treated me in a healthier way. Although I brought a destructive influence into his home, I felt loved and accepted and wasn't treated rudely or disrespectfully. When I acted rude and disrespectful, they attempted to communicate to me that my behavior was unacceptable, somehow always implying that I was acceptable. It was an important lesson for me to have experienced. But it was years before I looked back and consciously felt remorse for the chaos and upset I brought to my birth-father's family.

I finished high school on the honor roll. I was smoking in the smoking area, still enjoying my out-of-control eating and drinking. I was going dancing in night clubs, with a fake ID, four or five nights a week.

These early experiences and influences set up patterns that became real obstacles to happy, productive adult living. Looking back, I see that during those early years I began to establish unhealthy ways of relating to others and myself. Very early in my childhood, the pattern of almost complete repression of fear set in motion a style of high-risk behavior. As a teen, I adopted a style of appearing powerful, needless, fearless, opinionated. I used anger and charm alternatingly to intimidate and manipulate others. It always looked as if I were strong and they were weak, as if they were dependent on me and I was independent. I believed it, they believed it.

During my twenties my weight started to go up and down; I always used diet pills to get it down. I married and had two children. I picked a husband who was emotionally dependent on me. He had early childhood abandonment issues and drank in an obsessive, compulsive way. I felt secure—my own drinking and eating looked OK in comparison. I unconsciously used him to reinforce my denial about the severity of my own eating and drinking. I focused on him in many ways to defuse the pain of looking at me. Only much later did I discover that it's very common for an adult child of an alcoholic to marry an alcoholic.

My husband began to show signs of chronic alcoholism in his late twenties. By his early thirties, serious physical symptoms began to appear. The heartbreak of being powerless to stop his downward cycle, combined with my abuse of diet pills, overeating and drinking, made coping with life next to impossible.

I lost my natural optimism about life. I was incapable of emotionally supporting my children. Even with the best of intentions, I had nevertheless become the most dreaded thing I could imagine—*I had become my mother.* When I realized I was a woman unable to be a good parent, I hit an emotional bottom. A pit so deep I thought I might not be able to climb out.

The arrival of my twenty-ninth birthday found me overweight, riddled with feelings of failure and still struggling to present a picture of perfection to the world. Each day, through my thoughts and behaviors, I helplessly added to my self-hate, anger, resentment and hopelessness. In desperation, I made a call to an organization specializing in the education and treatment of alcoholism—for him.

, A spark of hope came wrapped in the package of information about alcoholism—its genetic predisposition, its incurable, progressive and fatal nature and *how it affects all the members of the family.* I discovered I wasn't alone in this experience and I didn't need to place blame. They told me, "You didn't cause it, you can't control it, and you can't cure it." They explained about recovery, about arresting alcoholism. Hope, at last. Pain mixed with hope is a totally different experience from hopeless pain.

I had found direction for alcoholism recovery and the guidance to address the unhealthy relationship issues that were plaguing my life. It was suggested that I seek out local self-help groups, groups using the 12-Step solution.

I intuitively knew that this information about the addictive disease process could also apply to my eating problem. Recovery from an addictive disease, I learned, had to happen on a physical, mental, emotional and spiritual level. My excitement grew as I began to see how to apply this information to both my eating and drinking.

I also began to see how my relationship and control issues got enmeshed with the eating disorder compulsion and obsessions. I saw how I used my body shape and weight to sometimes push people away and other times to pull them closer. I became aware of my history of using my body image to define and manipulate my self-esteem.

Now, not only was I willing to go to any length to stay sober and to abstain from random, compulsive overeating, I was willing to look at all the old beliefs that had kept me tied to unhealthy relationships.

Even though I was beginning to feel better than I ever had, things got worse. I watched my husband and my children struggle with the changes in the family and the changes in me. When I had 21 days of abstinence from eating in between meals, my husband was hospitalized because of his drinking problem and almost died. The children were just six and three, and although I wasn't able to offer an abundance of support and understanding in our home, I continued to abstain, no matter what.

When I had 30 days of abstinence, my step-father had a stroke. Again, I didn't use my eating disorder to deal with life's stress. I didn't break my abstinence. I knew that random, compulsive overeating would make any situation worse and I didn't have the strength to live though "worse."

While I had chosen recovery, my husband struggled with his own life and death issues. I came to the conclusion that a separation would offer me the drug and alcohol free home that the children and I deserved. In my heart, I felt my husband was choosing death when he began to drink again, and I believed that the kids and I had the right to not watch him slowly die at close range any longer.

I remember watching him pack up the last of his things and as he drove away, I thought it might be the last time I would see him alive. I knew he had the right to choose to live or die and I knew I had the right to choose to not watch, but the sadness was engulfing! Sadness for those two young lovers who had lost their dreams and their way; sadness for our children who lost out on a healthy, stable, supportive home that had both a mother and a father.

To my surprise, within 60 days of moving out of the house, he made a commitment to sobriety—to live. Although the marriage was over, we both have continued to honor our commitment to recovery.

Now with new tools for living, I deepened my commitment to being the type of parent I could admire. I stayed abstinent and sober. I took classes, read books and regularly went to an open forum at a local university that offered counseling and advice for families in need of help.

In those first few years, I stumbled along, discovering many realities about me and my world. I took workshops, seminars and immersed myself in self-help groups. They offered me insight into the rhyme and rhythm of how I got to be who I was and the key to understanding how to change and grow into the person I'd like to be.

I developed a style of meditating that opened the door to a wonderful internal world. Through visualizations, I discovered an inner family of "past Beckys" who needed re-parenting, acceptance, guidance and forgiveness. I began building loving, functional relationships with this inner family. I also discovered older, wiser inner selves who brought experience and more recovery to this magical inner family. Working with this new found "family" provided healing of my past experiences, past interpretations and attitudes—a healing of my past.

In those first few years, there were many days when I had to walk through difficult, fearful experiences, but I had finally grown to the point where the pain of **not** walking through a difficult situation was greater than the pain of putting one foot in front of the other and just trudging through them. There were tears of sadness, tears of anger and rage, and tears of joy. There was fun and lightness in my living I never would have imagined. I went back to school and acquired a healthy ambition to learn and an interest in adding to life. I was becoming a woman I liked.

After a few years of recovery, I discovered a lump in my breast. After the shock, I sat still and evaluated my life from yet another perspective. I asked myself some important questions: Do the people I love **know** I love them? Do I have any amends to others that haven't been made? If I had only 18 months to live, is there anything I would want to do or accomplish? Attempting to answer these questions brought my life to a new level of living. The quality of my life increased as I began to live each day as if it were one of my last.

Because of the lump in my breast, I began to change the way I nourished myself, and my family. I realized that even though I was abstaining, meaning I didn't eat in between meals, I didn't eat very healthy at those meals. I changed majors at school and made nutrition my graduate level focus. I drastically reduced the fats and oils in my diet. I read labels and didn't purchase chemical-laden foods. I did a daily meditation that included amends to my body. I apologized to my body for not knowing how to take better care of it. I re-committed myself to developing a better understanding and communication with my body.

I gathered a supportive team of health professionals. After awhile the lump became cyclical and gradually disappeared. The lump, which initially seemed like a tragedy, became one of the best things to ever happen to me.

After about six years of recovery, I was given the opportunity to work in the field of recovery, first, with recovery from alcoholism, then with children of alcoholics and finally with recovery from eating disorders.

I always knew my problem was with eating, not weight, so when the phrase "eating disorders" started appearing in every day society, I identified. I wasn't a vomiter, I didn't relate to the starving to be underweight and I didn't relate to chronic dieting. My uncontrollable eating created a pattern of gradual weight gain followed by severe restricting through the magic of diet pills. My eating disorder was the classic yo-yo weight syndrome—out of control eating equalled weight gain and temporary control measures meant weight loss. The cycle meant insanity.

I knew I had a eating disorder even though my all-too-common pattern wasn't being labeled as an eating disorder. I knew that I'd found a permanent solution. The constant, mind-nagging chatter about weight, weight loss, body judging, body rejection—the obsessive, compulsive relationship with food, eating, weight, shape and size—was **gone.** I hadn't just "gotten better," I was experiencing recovery.

One of the most rewarding projects, both professionally and personally, was being part of a committee that started a residential center for people with eating disorders. I became the executive director and designed and implemented an exciting program. I lectured at universities, hospitals and clinics. The medical and clinical communities are uniformly a committed group and were always supportive and excited about the information I presented.

Getting to see residents who were on the verge of death or insanity begin to recover was an experience I can't adequately describe. The experience gave me an opportunity to re-honor my own recovery and cherish that special kind of love that heals.

With the arrival of my forties, I've looked back and seen the changes that happened as I stumbled along. One of the most enjoyable successes has been that since 1974, I have abstained from compulsive eating and maintained a stable, healthy body weight. I have achieved a charmed attitude, although not a charmed life.

I can't emphasize enough my belief that the Overeaters Anonymous 12 Steps, literature, fellowship and meetings can offer the understanding and long term support essential to the pursuit of recovery.

My purpose for this book is to help provide you with a way to live without the dominating insanity of any and all expressions of eating disorders, to offer you tools and insights that can bring increased self-acceptance and self-love. My hope is to ignite in you a "knowing" that the freedom to live and dream can be yours, again.

YOU CAN'T GET THERE FROM HERE

Margo C.

[Margo C. is 40 years old and has three years of abstinence from compulsive eating. She is a healthy looking, athletic woman who does mountain climbing and hiking for recreation. Margo sees hints of her eating disorder in childhood behavior.]

I started hiding food, which would indicate to me that I knew something was wrong. I was probably 10 or 11. The clearest memory I have is I used to love potato chips and dip made with blue cheese, onion juice and milk. I would go through a whole pound of blue cheese and a bag of potato chips. Then I'd hide the empty bag under my bed until I had a chance to get it to a place where no one would know what I'd done. I did a lot of sneaky eating. I just knew I didn't want people to know what I was doing. Inherent in that is the knowledge at some level that there was something wrong with my eating.

I remember when I was in college, the snack bar closed at night and I got to the point where I would go and get two BLT's, a hamburger and two orders of french fries and a bunch of candy because I couldn't stand going back to the dorm without it, and I was real embarrassed by that.

I tried to diet more times than I care to tell you and was never very successful at dieting. A lot of people with this disease dieted real well. I never dieted well.

I felt shame. Oh God, so much shame. If I were a good person, if I were a strong person, I would be able to control this. If I only had the discipline inside. Those words came from my family and I bought into them real well. If I were a disciplined, strong, self-willed, together person, I would simply say "No I'm not going to eat it." Boy, I believed that 100%.

I bounced back and forth between being very rigid and controlled about what I ate for a few days and then letting it go for two or three days, and then being very rigid and controlled for a few days and then losing it for two or three days. The sense of "I'll be a good girl for two or three days and then I can do whatever I want for a couple of days." It was like the four to five days of "goodness" and the two days of "badness" started to change places. The days that I could maintain the "goodness" became less and the days that I felt like I could eat whatever I wanted became more.

I got out of school and went to work in an accounting office. I was 22 at that point. That's when the control started to shift. The number of days that I could be *good* started to shrink and the number of days that I had to be *bad* grew. My drinking also increased during this time. The two seemed to go hand in hand.

I started gaining weight. When I got out of college I weighed probably 120. By the time I moved to Aspen I was 25 so it was about three and a half years later and I weighed 175. It happened slowly and gradually. I was still active physically. I was still playing softball and I was still playing volleyball and doing that kind of stuff. I was in and out of relationships. But definitely the control was just gone.

It was very clear in my head, "good/bad" eating meant "good/bad" girl. They went together. There was no separation between the way I ate and who I was. The way I ate was how I felt about myself. I felt worthless, basically. How could you respect someone who was fat? If I couldn't have at least enough discipline to not eat like a pig, how could I have respect for myself? I didn't.

[Margo got involved with EST training while living in Aspen, Colorado, and her obsession with that relieved her obsession with eating. At about 26, she began doing cocaine and lost a great deal of weight, ending up at 103 pounds and wearing a size two dress.]

I moved to Aspen weighing 175 pounds. I took the EST training and eight months later I weighed 125. It was effortless. There was no obsession with food. There was no dieting, I just ate less. I was obsessed with EST. In a sense that was a way of controlling my eating. I got obsessed with being on the staff at EST training. I worked 11 hours a day six days a week and I never had time to eat. Food wasn't a big deal. It was not about dieting. I just got to the end of eight months and I was thin.

I discovered cocaine at 26 or 27. At first it was very social coke use, but probably two years later, I got into doing lines and got very thin—I weighed 102 or 103 which for me is very, very thin. I loved it. I also at that point I was doing a lot of drugs. That five year period (ages 25-30) was a very heavy drug use period. When I moved to Aspen, on the first day I was there, my sister gave me my first hit of acid. I did a lot of hallucinogenics. I did a lot of cocaine. I smoked pot on a daily basis for five years. Most of that was really fun—I was not yet at a point where my life was awful.

Food wasn't an issue. It just really wasn't. But very clearly the drugs took the focus off the food so **they** were a controlling issue without my being aware that that was going on.

Weight-wise I got to the place where I'd always told myself, if only I looked like this, if only I were this thin, then everything would be fine. I had a great body. I was in the best shape of my life and I was miserable. So the one thing that I pinned my hopes on didn't happen. I was unhappier than I was aware of being at any time in my life.

The cocaine use got to be very addictive and very destructive the last year I was there. I had begun to steal drugs from my roommates. I stole drugs from my dealer. Oh God, there was real shame attached to this one.

Having the drugs was more important than any kind of ethics I had. It just made my own sense of "you have no self-discipline, you're not worth anything, you're not worthy of anybody's respect" get much worse.

I was also isolating. Yes, I skied and yes, I played tennis but I wasn't functionally social. I hated that I wanted to be alone, that I didn't want to be with people. I felt very torn. It felt like too much trouble to be out there in the world and yet I didn't like being by myself.

[At about 30 years of age, Margo moved to New York. She continued isolating and started to gain weight again.]

I thought the move would "fix" it. That I'd get away from the drugs. That I'd get a serious job. I worked the whole time I was in Aspen but it wasn't the nine to five, professional, Madison Avenue kind of job that I had grown up believing success was about. So I figured, I've had my fun, I've had my fling with drugs. I'll get away from the drugs. I'll go find a great job and a great apartment in New York and be a professional and be successful.

When I moved back to New York, I was a size two. I was very thin but I couldn't figure out why I wasn't happy. I tried to control my eating but it only worked for maybe one meal at a time. I gained 80 pounds in about a year and a half.

I weighed 180 pounds and was doing $1,000 a week worth of cocaine; it didn't stop the eating anymore. I did cocaine to escape the pain and the horrendous feelings around looking like what I was starting to look like.

At that point, I started not being able to get to work. I was doing a computer job and I started taking a computer home. Everything was too much trouble. Everything was too hard. Getting from my apartment to the office was too much of a project for me to deal with.

Having to write a program that was technically difficult was too much for me to deal with. It was not OK for me to make *any* kind of mistake at that point. My priorities, my proportions got all screwed up. At this point I had so little self-esteem that any little mistake was so huge I stopped doing anything.

I finally quit my job. I made up all kinds of rational reasons why the job was not right for me. I didn't work for about three or four months. In Aspen, I did drugs with other people. In New York I did cocaine by myself.

During that time, my mom offered to send me a "fat farm." I was in tears at her house one day about this weight thing. She said delicately, "Have you ever thought about a fat farm?" I said yes I had but I couldn't afford to go. She didn't know that the reason I didn't have any money was because I was putting it all in drugs. She said "What if I pay for it?" So she sent me to a spa.

I was there for eight weeks. I lost 25 pounds. This is one of those places where if you don't have an eating disorder, it's great. It taught all the right things to do. For the first time in my life someone did some behavior work and did some therapy work and said this is what you can do and you can take this home with you. It was about moderate exercise and moderate eating. It wasn't about dieting, it was about moderate. I said all right, but just like people with eating disorders, I couldn't do any of it. I mean I just couldn't do it.

[Margo's cocaine use decreased after her eight-week stay at the spa, but she discovered laxatives.]

I lost 25 pounds at the spa and I also discovered that I weighed less when I took laxatives. I got constipated and took a laxative. Then somebody said if one doesn't work right, take a couple. So I took a couple and my face looked thinner to me. I thought, hmmmmmm.

It took about six months to begin taking them when they weren't necessary. Six months later I was maybe doing two or three laxatives once a week, not indicated, just doing it. Also, it made me feel emptier. It began to build up and I can't tell you how that happened. I have looked and I've meditated and I've written trying to discover how it happened but I don't know how I got from two or three laxatives once or twice a week to taking **between 50-90 a day five days a week.**

My body wouldn't tolerate any more than that. There were physical symptoms, emotional symptoms, and also, my drinking escalated.

Doing about 50 laxatives a day, three or four days a week, I got down to 131 pounds. My knuckles were so white they looked like a skeleton. I was beginning to have weakness symptoms then and they just increased as the numbers of laxatives increased. The isolation increased and my ability to function decreased.

I got real aware of hating myself. Absolute self-hatred. Looking back, it's the first time it was real clear that it was self-hatred. I couldn't stand me.

I was in the middle of this incredible laxative abuse where I couldn't even walk up the stairs without cramping, the physical symptoms got really awful.

I had an alcoholic sister who ended up in treatment in Tucson and I went out to her "family week." I thought I was out there to fix my sister, but the first night I was there they told us, you're not here for your patient, you're here for you. My stomach fell through the floor.

They asked us to share what some of our goals were for that week. I went first and shared some goals I thought they wanted to hear. Then three or four more people shared and my hand went up again. I say it went up because I didn't put it up. I said I need to tell you all that I abuse laxatives and one of my goals is to not. I had never told anybody that. I'd told my therapist and I'd told my mother, period. Nobody else knew about that. I was deathly ashamed and I shared it with all these people.

They talked about the first Step (of the 12 Steps) that night, the powerlessness. They talked about a *God concept.* They talked about you don't ever have to be alone. And I was like a sponge.

Four days later someone came within six inches of my face and said, **"You have an eating disorder and it's primary, progressive and fatal, and with the information you've given us about your heart, you've got about six months to live."** They handed me a card for an eating disorder treatment center. I called them that afternoon and I was in treatment ten days later.

I was so relieved. I was so happy. I was so glad someone could say you're not weak, you're not awful, you're not undeserving of respect, you're not undisciplined, you have a **disease.** You have an illness. It's not your fault and you're not alone. I was relieved, hopeful, delighted, ecstatic and terrified.

The wonderful thing for me was a God concept. I mean the whole idea of having a God in my life and I don't have to do it by myself was wonderful. The days when I get up and I say I don't have a clue how to even put my clothes on are the days when my life works the best. It's called a surrender to a Higher Power. I got that from day one, from the first day I walked into the codependency program at the other treatment center. I got that—I got a God concept.

Working a 12-Step program is doing footwork. It's about a *bottom line*. I sometimes forget to talk about that, but the bottom line is that I don't eat between meals, no matter what. That's the bottom line. Without that I have no life. I had no life when I came in to recovery. Emotionally I just wasn't alive. For me, God came first and then abstinence came.

You don't eat in between meals, no matter what. I mean, that's got to be first. You don't eat no matter what. If it takes quitting your job, if it takes leaving your husband, I don't care what it takes. You don't eat between meals, no matter what.

And you work with a sponsor. You work with someone who's a "winner." You work with someone who's got some time abstinent, who's got a life that you like, and you listen and do what you're told. You do what you're told whether you like it or you understand it, you just do it in the beginning.

After about 10 months of abstinence, I went into therapy. My own belief around eating disorders is that you've got to be abstinent. I don't know anybody with an eating disorder who doesn't need clinical support—therapy, but unless you're abstinent, therapy is worthless. In New York I had had therapy for five years.

Family of origin issues were the biggest ones. The two issues that I went to therapy for this time were my mother and intimacy. They are painful issues, both of them. I don't know of any compulsive overeaters who are not codependent.

But you've got to get abstinent first. Until I had abstinence, my brain, nothing functioned. I couldn't hear any of the rest of this stuff. But I also believe that without dealing with the intimacy, the codependency, the family of origin issues, that the chances of staying abstinent just get smaller and smaller and smaller.

Don't ever give up. I see a lot of people around who just don't get it. They keep trying and they keep trying and they keep trying and don't give up. There is always hope out there. The tools are there and it's about not giving up.

I share with people who are brand new that abstinence is not about specifically what you put in your mouth, it's about you just eat three times a day, period. What you choose to eat during those three times a day is about health and is about moderation. What I tell them is for right now, get abstinent and we'll deal with the food later. We'll deal with if you're eating healthy later. I couldn't, and I don't think anybody can, deal with health issues until you've got some abstinence under your belt and can start being a sane person.

I have dreams. I didn't have any dreams when I got here. I couldn't let myself dream because I knew I couldn't do it. I believe today that I can do stuff, maybe not all at once. I'm learning to do things not because I think I should. I look at what I want to do and ask, is it going to hurt anybody and is it going to hurt me? If the answers to those questions are no, I go for it.

I'm learning to listen to my gut to find out what I want. And that isn't, "I want two pieces of cake and eight pies," that's not the want I'm talking about. I'm talking about want from a nurturing place, from a fulfilling place. There's a really clear difference between what I want and what my disease wants.

I learned somewhere incorrectly that all of my feelings were extreme and inappropriate. What I've been given is the knowledge that that's not true. My feelings are OK, and by making them OK, my feelings are much less extreme and inappropriate! I can just be who I am and know in my heart that I'm a worthwhile human being today.

NEVER LOSE HOPE

Jeanie M.

[Jeanie is working toward a Ph.D. in English literature. She's 46 years old, has been married about 25 years, and has two grown children. Jeanie has been in Overeaters Anonymous for about 15 years but just recently celebrated two years of continuous abstinence. Her earliest childhood memories suggest an odd relationship with food and eating.]

My parents described me as an "under-eater" when I was little. I remember being finicky, and I certainly got the message I was not eating enough. My first memory of compulsive overeating was when I was six years old and ate a whole box of chocolate candy. I broke out in hives and wasn't able to go to the Christmas program.

I started gaining weight when I was about seven or eight. At school kids began teasing me about being fat. I remember when I was eight and in the third grade, we were all weighed by the school nurse. I was standing in line praying that my weight would be under 100 pounds and, whatever it was, that she would say it quietly. Everybody else was weighing around 60 to 80 pounds. I don't think anyone was even 90. I remember standing there praying and the nurse just boomed it out, "103 pounds!" Everybody down the line was saying, "Oh my God, Jeanie weighs 103 pounds, 103 pounds, 103 pounds." It was so painful.

At that time, I began to notice that I looked different, that clothes looked different on me than they did on other people. I had to go into the chubby section to buy dresses when I was eight or nine. The salesladies would sometimes make remarks about my weight and I felt absolutely humiliated. I also felt surprised that someone would comment on my body. The pain I felt was compounded by the fact that when I had been much younger, I had gotten lots of strokes for being a really cute little girl—even winning a beauty contest at four years old. Not receiving that kind of praise anymore, but going on with the illusion that I was exceptionally pretty, I was really surprised and hurt that people didn't treat me in a special way anymore.

Even as a child, I guess I knew that if you ate too much, you got fat, but somehow the connection didn't work for me because I was still operating on the idea that I should finish everything on my plate. One time, when I was about ten, I went out to eat and I ordered a steak dinner. The waitress said, "Oh, I'm sure you won't be able to eat all that." I remember saying with pride, "Oh yes I will! I'll be able to eat all of that." I felt like I was doing something good to eat a whole adult meal.

I think I got a lot of mixed messages about food and eating. There were times when people really let me indulge myself, and I would eat lots of food—maybe three hamburgers at once. At other times, people told me, "Don't pick at that," or "That'll make you fat," or "Don't eat that."

When I was ten years old, I went to a fair in our city. There was a woman there, handing out samples of skim milk which was a new item in our stores in the Midwest. The woman was very slim, but in the background there was a huge blow-up picture of her the way she had been—she had weighed over 300 pounds. I remember that it absolutely blew my mind that this woman had actually lost all that weight. It just seemed incredible to me that someone could actually change themselves so drastically. I had just started getting the idea that God had chosen for me to be fat—that I was somehow condemned to being fat. Now all of a sudden, I had an awareness that people could lose weight and fat people could be thin. I remember talking to my mother about that. Actually, the outcome of that event was that my mother wrote the woman a letter to ask how she had lost her weight. The woman wrote back with a letter and her diet. My mother only told me about the diet; she didn't tell me about the letter. I found the letter later. It said something like, "Oh yes, I know you must be very concerned about your little fatty." I remember burning with shame when I read those words.

Evidently the "skim milk" diet didn't work. My mother knew how unhappy I was, and when I was eleven, she took me to the doctor and I went on a diet. The doctor was very opposed to diet pills. He told me never, never to take them and tried to impress me with how damaging they could be to my body. I should have remembered that later on. He was very sympathetic and kind to me; he had a teen-aged daughter who had the same problem I did. His plan seems simple now, but at the time his ideas were new to me: he gave me a list of foods to eat and not to eat. He told me to write down everything I ate each day and count the calories. I had to make sure that I was under 1200 calories per day and then report to him each month. By this time, at age eleven, I weighed 130 pounds.

Over a period of months I lost weight. One day I came home after a dance class and got on the scale; I weighed 99 pounds. It was the first time I had weighed under 100 pounds since I was seven years old.

Through my teenage years, I gained a little bit of weight. Every day of my life I was on a diet—or at least each day I would start out that way. I wasn't terribly overweight, but most of the time I had a fifteen pound cushion and I played with that weight, although it wasn't really play. Recently though, I visited a friend I had known since high school. She was surprised when I was talking about how hard it was for me in high school and what body image problems I had. She said, "I never thought of you as being overweight in high school. I never really noticed that until college." But I remember comments from boys from time to time.

In college I weighed about 142 pounds. I'm five six and a half, so that's not a significantly high weight for my height. But I felt overweight. I came from the Midwest to go to college in California. You could get by in the Midwest being fifteen pounds overweight; in California there was much more emphasis on body size. I can remember people treating me a different way in college, as if I were very overweight.

When I was about 20, I discovered diet pills. I went to a diet doctor—interestingly, a very overweight doctor. He gave me a prescription for diet pills. I had a terrible physical reaction to the pills: not sleeping the whole first night, not sleeping much of the second night, waking up hallucinating, feeling my legs trembling, and then losing the feeling in my legs—all sorts of problems. By the third day I had begun to recover somewhat from the reaction, so I took another pill. I continued to take pills until my body almost adjusted to them. I was still hardly sleeping at all and was very nervous most of the time. I continued the pills in spite of the physical reaction for one reason: I was really desperate to be thin. I remember fully knowing those pills were damaging my health and probably my brain, but I took them anyway because they were the first things in my life that made me not want to eat.

I did lose weight on the pills—down to about 117 pounds. I was 21 and thin, but it was an unhappy time in my life. A close friend of mine had died, I had broken up a long-term relationship, and I was really depressed, but I kept taking the pills because I wanted to lose just a little more. I wanted to be 115. That was my ideal weight.

Before I could lose those last pounds, I began to feel the effects of not being able to sleep. My answer was to start drinking a six-pack of beer every night. I'd wake in the morning and take a pill, then that night drink a six-pack of beer. The calories from the beer were almost the only ones I was taking in, but I started gaining weight at that time. Since I was going home for a month before I came back for my senior year, I decided I would use that time to stop the pills and stop drinking and just try to equalize and stay at the weight I was. But when I started gaining weight, I couldn't control it.

In November of that year, I met the man who was to become my husband—I weighed 125 pounds, but by the time we got married the following summer, I was up to 150 pounds. I just continued to gain weight in spite of trying to control it.

In my twenties I tried lots of things to lose weight like Weight Watchers, gyms, diets of all kinds. When I had my children I gained way too much weight; then after they were born I tried to diet it off. I even took shots. The doctor injected me with the placenta of a sheep, or something like that. I don't know what they were, but they were so expensive I thought the cost would keep me on the diet—I imagined that I wouldn't be able to bear to go off the diet after spending that kind of money. But I found that the money made no difference.

I had joined Weight Watchers probably, in truth, fifteen different times. I got acquainted with the lecturers and clerks at lots of different meetings. I remember one clerk at Weight Watchers asking me, "How many times are you going to join?" I said, "This is the last time. The next time I'll just commit suicide." I kind of said "Ha ha ha," but it wasn't funny—I didn't know any other place to go.

I remember quitting Weight Watchers for the last time—quitting everything and then just bingeing the whole winter. I had stopped smoking and had gained a lot of weight. In fact, I was the heaviest I'd ever been in my life—I weighed 188 pounds. I was 31 years old.

I outweighed my husband. That number on the scale really hit me. I had come to an impasse. I knew I couldn't live any longer eating the way I was eating. It was just too painful to be 31, weigh 188 pounds and wear a muu-muu all the time. I wanted to die, but I knew I couldn't die with children depending on me. When you can't live and you can't die there isn't much of an alternative.

At that time, a good friend of mine said to me, and I really bless her for this now, "Why don't you try another group where you don't know anyone? I don't mean another Weight Watchers group—I mean another group."

I had read about Overeaters Anonymous some months before, but I thought all groups were the same, and my attitude was not the best. I thought that I would just go to a different place to fail again, but it wouldn't be so embarrassing since I didn't know as many people there, and everyone who was concerned about me would be satisfied I was doing something. I would go through the motions, but I had no hope that it would really work.

I really didn't understand my first meeting—all I heard was people sharing their experiences. I thought this was just the meeting where they were telling what happened to them, and that I must have to go to a different meeting to find out what it really was—how to do "the program." I thought there must be some kind of a secret meeting. On the O.A. directory, I saw an "old-timers" meeting listed and I thought, "Oh, that must be it—that must be where you go to find out the real secret of how to do it because these people are just telling what happened." I remember asking one woman questions and she said "Just work the Steps." I looked at the Steps and then felt completely disappointed. I thought they were ridiculous and I didn't want anything to do with the God part. In my opinion, believing in God was juvenile and actually stupid.

At my first meetings, however, I did hear people with insight into themselves. They were taking the whole matter seriously, and I believed that I had a serious disease. When they said the words, "compulsive overeater" I felt a relief. I thought, "Oh my God, that's what I am." I knew I wanted the insight that these people had, although I thought it was weird that these people talked so much about God.

At the end of my first meeting, I tried again to ask people questions. One woman told me, "Just keep coming back. Don't worry that you don't understand it. Just know that if you feel absolutely hopeless and desperate, you're in the right place." I felt at that moment a minor miracle had occurred since those were the exact two words I had used to describe how I felt before I had come; hopeless and desperate. I knew I was in the right place.

I came back the next week. I decided that I was going to be committed to going to this, certainly not to do any Steps, but just to **go** to the best diet club I'd ever found. I made a commitment that night I would abstain.

At that time in O.A., abstinence meant following a very rigid "food plan." I started following it on my own, but one night I was approached by a woman who was new at sponsoring and who wanted some people to sponsor. Although I really didn't want her as a sponsor, I didn't have enough self confidence to say no. I said, "Oh, OK, I am looking for a sponsor." But I said that I could see that the questions that she wanted me to write on were designed to lead to some sort of spiritual experience. I told her I didn't want her to be disappointed because I wasn't going to have one.

I found out later these writings were questions from another organization not affiliated with O.A. There were 30-day assignments, and by the end of the 30 days I did have a spiritual experience. I had had a traditional sort of Protestant upbringing and had believed in God, but had drifted off from religion and really didn't want it in my life. At that time I was reading a lot of yoga books, and these helped me to be able to identify with a universal life force, but I had a hard time separating spirituality from religion. I thought that in order to work the steps of O.A. I had to believe in the God of my childhood and all the dogma that went it. When I was reading these books on Eastern religion, I got in touch with the idea of a universal life force and the idea of a God within all of us and within plants and every living thing. Philosophically, I was able to accept that life force. Once I was able to accept that, a lot of things fell into place. Today I can say "God" but at that time I could only say "Higher Power"—but it was a beginning.

Once started, I lost a lot of weight—71 pounds. *But then I found I couldn't move from the weight-loss food plan into a comfortable maintenance abstinence.* When I would start gaining a little bit of weight, instead of just seeing that as a fluctuation and feeling comfortable with what I was doing, I would panic. I would think that I was violating something—that I had done something wrong and I was gaining weight. So I'd say to myself, "I'm going to have to go back on the weight-loss food plan until I lose this weight, and then I can resume the maintenance." I would try to go back on it, but I found I couldn't do it. I was too depleted. I got into a cycle of trying to find a comfortable "food plan" for maintenance, putting on weight and trying to go back to the weight-loss food plan; then the cycle would start over again. As I was going along, I was gaining a little bit of weight, a little bit of weight, a little bit of weight.

In 1979, after I'd been abstaining for about four and a half years, my dad died. I was pretty much bingeing instead of eating meals when I was home for the funeral. I mark that point as the beginning of my physical relapse. It was the beginning of a long downhill road. I never quit going to O.A., although there were times when I would go for months without going to a meeting. But if you asked me if I was in O.A., I'd say yes. I never tried anything else because I knew somehow the answers were here for me, but I just didn't know what to do. I'd used all the tools, I'd given service, I'd sponsored lots of people, and I still couldn't get a comfortable abstinence.

Abstinence was a food plan—that's the concept I had. I was aware of two factions in the program at that time. One group said there was no way that you could eat white flour or sugar and even function. That school of thought maintained that those were the only two addictive foods. **After having gained back over 80 pounds without eating them, I realized that it was not just about those two foods.** The other faction said just walk a God-centered path, work the Steps, and then your abstinence will come. Do all that you're supposed to do and your abstinence will come naturally and your weight will drop off. From 1979 to 1984, I was just going back and forth and back and forth between the two different factions.

I felt like there was absolutely no place to go. I had run the gamut in O.A. I felt as though I knew what there was to do—I knew all about O.A. and what to do, but I just couldn't do it. I was back to feeling suicidal again—the exact same way I felt when I had first come to O.A. I was hopeless, I was desperate—only this time I was in O.A. I didn't want to live and I didn't really want to choose to die. Here I was: I hadn't eaten sugar for 12 years and I had a weight gain of over 80 pounds. It felt like the end of the road.

Then I found out about a new residential center in town that used the 12 Steps—a recovery home for people with eating disorders. They had a non-residential program and, without much hope, I went in for a screening. I began with the idea that I knew everything—that I knew what to do but just somehow wasn't able to do it. I found that that wasn't true. I got a lot of information about eating disorders that was entirely new to me.

This new information meant hope, but you have to realize I was pretty cynical and I was not sure anything was going to help. I was especially worried about eating different foods. I had come in convinced that sugar was my main addiction, but I couldn't figure out why I'd gained all the weight back. I thought I was just going to be devastated by eating sugar. I truly thought I might have a physical and emotional reaction (go crazy and have palpitations or something the first time I ate it). That didn't happen.

In fact, I began to take in lots of new concepts that helped me. First, I got the structure of three meals a day, eating moderately and knowing in my heart what was moderate. I became aware that I wasn't addicted to foods in particular. Actually, including all foods in my absti- nence and not restricting any foods was a release of the dieting mentality for me—*I had never given that up. I thought I had, but I hadn't. I fully understood for the first time that I had an eating disorder.*

One of the major things that I learned was that I truly have a disease. On some level, I had understood this concept in O.A. before, but I hadn't understood it to the very depth of my being or to the very depths of the disease. I had thought that an eating disorder was an emotional disease, and that if I got enough emotional health or enough spiritual health, then the disease wouldn't be active. Now I understand that I have an addictive disease—I didn't cause it, I can't control it and I can't cure it. There is a lot of surrender in that realization.

I had to separate my *feelings* from my *abstinence*. I had to make a commitment to abstain, no matter what, so that I could handle my emotional issues—not through eating bigger meals and not through bingeing or using my feelings as a reason to break my abstinence. I now believe there is no excuse that justifies returning to an active disease.

One of the most important things I've learned is that part of recovery is a process of relearning how to live with food and relating to food for the rest of my life. I had never really let go of the fear that I might overeat sometime again. Now I don't have that fear. I know, in my heart, that I don't have to be afraid inside. I have no mental reservation that I might—I don't feel that at all. I also think it's important to surround yourself with people who have an understanding of eating disorders so that you begin to lose the dieting mentality that we all come in with. **Perhaps most important of all, I believe that we must base recovery around not eating in between meals, rather than on a limited food plan.**

I feel, having survived all I've been through, I'm fortunate that I'm still around. I feel really lucky that I just didn't quit. It took me a long time to find the answers that I needed, but it was worth hanging around and worth all the pain. I can't even imagine what my life would be now if I were still out there eating. The wait was worth it.

BEAUTY AND BRAINS COULDN'T STOP IT

Lisa M.

[Lisa is 23 years old. She graduated from college a year ago with a degree in English literature, a minor in journalism and a theater emphasis as well. She worked at a Shakespearean theater all through college. Lisa celebrated her fourth abstinence birthday a few months ago. She recalls when she first became conscious of an odd relationship with eating.]

When I was very young, I remember my sister said, It's so hot, it's just too hot to eat." I said, "We could eat ice cream." I knew it was never too hot to eat. I also remember feeling different from the kids at school. Feeling like I was focused on food, almost more attached to it. I couldn't wait for lunch and I remember being really excited about dinner.

I didn't have a weight problem when I was little but I do remember having a weird body image thing when I was about eight or so. I rode the bus home, I had on a pair of shorts and I looked down at my legs. You know how when you sit down your thighs spread out. Well, I freaked out and thought I was fat. I ran home crying I was fat, I was fat. I remember talking to my parents and them saying, "No, you're not fat. Everyone's legs do that when you sit down." I think I had picked up a lot of body image stuff already at that age. I had already some inbred fear of being fat.

My mom struggled with a weight problem. I remember her asking me, at one point, something like "Are you embarrassed of me being overweight when I come to your school?" I remember that question really surprised me and I thought, "How could you think that I would be embarrassed?" I hadn't ever even thought of it, but on the other hand, at some level I was aware of it because I felt her pain. I was very, very connected to her eating problem. When she first found help for her eating disorder, I remember touching her and saying, "It's going to be OK, I know it's going to be OK."

[Lisa's mom started attending Overeaters Anonymous meetings when Lisa was about nine.]

I remember one time, I was really little, probably six or seven, I saw this woman on the street and she had on a halter top and hip-hugger bell-bottom jeans. She had a small waist and big hips. I said, "Oooh, when I grow up I want to look like that." Meaning, I wanted an hourglass figure—I thought that it was aesthetically pleasing. My mom and her friend said, "Oh no you don't," and "You're kidding, right?" I realized I liked the wrong thing—I didn't like what society likes. I wasn't really teased for liking it, just made to understand that this is not what we like. We don't like big hips.

I also remember being very different, always different. Feeling like I had this special case. I was a special child, I had special problems, special circumstances. I think I felt both bad and arrogant about that. I felt frustrated by it too because I think to a certain extent it was true. I was like a prodigy, I was reading by the time I was two. I was very mature and vocal and all that stuff. It wasn't like I was the only child like that, there were other kids too.

I guess it wasn't quite that bad when I was younger but by the time I got to junior high, it wasn't good. You got ostracized for getting good grades and working hard at school. I was just always worried about these things. I was scared that there was something wrong—like I didn't fit in. I had this part of me that knew I was OK but then I had this part of me that was always doubting it and worrying and looking around at the other kids to make sure that everything was going as it should, and that I wasn't wearing the wrong kind of shoes or saying the wrong kind of thing. That's what it was—I was self-obsessed from an early age!

I know my parents intended to impart all the right information. I know they really loved me but I think, especially with sexuality and all the body image things, I was picking up unresolved issues. The body image is a perfect example. I remember one time I said, "I'm pretty, I'm pretty." I was about three. My mom said, "Yes you are and it's healthy to know that." But then I kept saying it over and over and somebody told me I was conceited. I got very confused—why had somebody taken offense that I had said this about myself? I remember my mom explaining to me that it was perfectly OK to know that I'm pretty and it was healthy, but that for some reason other people don't like to hear you say it all the time. I think that's probably a really good thing to say to a child, but somehow I got mixed messages.

I used to think that what was wrong would be easier to pinpoint if I had parents who never said they loved me. Then I could say, "Aha, that's it, this is my problem!" but it's not true. It's taken me a long time to get it that, yes, I had really nice, loving parents and a real nice environment, but there were also a lot of things that were inappropriate and unhealthy. It's taken me a long time to see both sides. **The negative doesn't negate the positive**—it's OK to acknowledge the part that wasn't the way you'd paint it in your perfect ideal.

I think my difficulties were more about having this disease and how it affected the way I relate to myself. At this point though, it's good to remember and acknowledge my history. I feel like I've gotten through a lot of what I need to get through to feel comfortable with myself. It seemed so hard at the beginning and I'm sure there are other layers to be uncovered later, but it feels like a lot of that has been worked out with relative ease because I did have the knowledge that my parents loved me and supported me.

When I was 14, my grandfather died. We were in Kentucky dealing with all the grief and the funeral. Everyone had brought the traditional hordes of food over. It was the first time I remember having a bingeing experience.

I felt it was time to be the very responsible daughter and help out, be the fortitude, the pillar of strength, whatever. All I remember really, is standing in front of an open refrigerator eating out of this trifle bowl. It was the first time I remember eating like that. I remember feeling sick there, lethargic and sick. I felt abandoned because everyone else was into their own emotional stuff. I was almost 14 and I just didn't know what to do—I felt tremendous grief.

It was there I had the first weight gain. I remember my mom saying something about it. I'm sure she did it in a very loving way, but the fact that she said something indicated she was afraid. She told me later that she knew I had the disease but she somehow hoped that if I didn't get to a certain point it might be retractable. She hadn't really accepted in her heart that it was a disease—she thought somehow we could avoid it.

I remember her remark made me really mad and really hurt. There was a tremendous amount of shame. It was like, "Oh no, I'm in it. I've got it!" Pretty much from that point, I knew I was lost. I knew I was headed for O.A. I knew O.A. was about far more than just dieting but there was a part of me that took over for the rest of my high school years, trying to keep me in control.

I started dieting. I think I was trying to be sane about it and just kind of cut back on the quantities. I was trying to eat less or eat healthier. I know I thought sugar was *bad* so I would try not to eat sugar. I know for everything I cut out, I had to find something to fill it up, so I'm sure I drank a lot of diet sodas or chewed a lot of gum. It was very much trading off. I always found a way to get my fix.

At about 14 years old I started having really bad migraine

headaches. I really used them with my disease. I used them to stay home. I used them to get attention. I used them to explain away my problems, just like I would use food. We were all convinced that the headaches were because of *what* I ate. I had this whole hypoglycemic thing and this candida thing. All these diets I had to follow gave me a medical excuse to control. It didn't seem quite as sick because it was sanctioned by doctors. I'm sure that they didn't know that I was using three different diets that cancelled each other out and that I'd eat only tomatoes and lettuce because that was all that was left between the three diets. I'd do the restriction as long as I could, then I'd binge. But then it was like I've got to get back on this diet thing; if I could just eat this way for the rest of my life I wouldn't have headaches, I'd be thin, I wouldn't be unpopular. In reality though, I wasn't unpopular. I was never the cheerleader but I had friends and I had a boyfriend.

I knew that I was supposed to be the princess who got all the attention, who was the homecoming queen, who was the most beautiful, the most talented, the smartest. I knew I was supposed to be the ultimate in everything but the world was not responding. I thought it was because of my weight.

Going to college meant separating from the boyfriend I'd had for five years. I was pretty dependent on him, on my family and all my friends. I had had this feeling of being less-than and not quite part of the inner circle. I knew that I had not had the popularity that I wanted. So I went to college determined to be popular and live the college experience that I'd heard about. This was going to be my *moment*. This was where people would be smart enough to understand me.

For nine or ten weeks I was just wild. From the first moment I walked on campus I was eating. I had had a really controlled summer. I had dieted down and was very thin. I was feeling euphoria from being at that controlled weight. I remember the first day just being really fascinated by lunch.

I dated ten men in ten weeks, all overlapping, and manipulated them, pitting them against each other. Oh yeah, I'll go to the party with you, pick me up at eight. Oh yeah, I'll got to the party with you, pick me up at eight. Oh no, I'm mixed up. You're both here. Let's all go together. I'd act like nothing's wrong. I was really inappropriate and out-of-control and lying. It was crazy, crazy, crazy. I don't remember studying. I did really well, but I don't remember anything related to studying.

By Thanksgiving, I had gained weight and I'd had a lot of *men* disappointments. The controlling thing with these men wasn't working and some of them started turning their attention elsewhere—that panicked me. I thought, "I'm not good enough." I remember coming home, seeing my boyfriend and feeling embarrassed the first time with him. I'd never been embarrassed of my body but I had gained probably ten pounds and felt really embarrassed.

After that first moment of shame, I pretty much lost all control and ate. The girl who had been at every party was now huddled in the bathroom stall of the dorm eating the leftover lasagne from the dorm dinner.

It was so frightening to me. I thought it was so insane and crazy, silly almost. Like it's just food, it's only food. I was like a drug addict. I spent money I didn't have. I'd drive around in my car alone all the time, in the middle of the night. I'd wake up from these dazes. One of the worse memories I have is waking up out of a fog in a pancake house in a scary part of town. I thought, "What am I doing? It's three in the morning and I have no money." I was like a blackout eater. I'd never heard of such a thing.

I just hated myself. I could not stand to be inside my skin. I would try to kind of fool myself for awhile. This was when I would do my "acting" thing. I'd tell myself, "I'll go home for Christmas, I'll diet the whole time and I'll be thin by the time I get back to school. Enough of this weight thing! I will be thin by the time I get back."

I had gained more weight by the time the holidays were over. I was in a panic. I was nothing, I hated myself so much. I knew that it was not stopping. I knew more was coming.

I started abusing laxatives, like about 40 a day. I didn't do it for very long, I knew how crazy and horrible it was.

I felt abandoned by my friends. I'm sure I was isolating but the invitations to parties were not coming any more. People would say things like, "What are you doing for exercise?" that kind of thinly-veiled comment. I thought everyone hated me. I was suicidal. I thought I could not go on if this was the way life was.

I remember I went to one O.A. meeting during high school. I hated it and I hated the people. I thought it was weird. But now I was desperate, so right after New Year's, I decided to go to O.A. again. It was scary, it was so foreign, all these people were weird. I'd lie and say I was doing OK and I'd sit in the back of the room. I had no clothes except for two pairs of sweats and a shirt. Oh, I also had this one pair of overalls. I hated the pity too. I felt like people were pitying me and I hated them. For a while, I would either leave at the break or I would binge all the way there and binge all the way home.

I was definitely falling apart. We had a dorm slide show toward the end of the year. There I was, pictures of me 40 pounds ago, at the beginning of the year. I laughed, but I was devastated. I moved out of my dorm and lived on the floor of a friend's, sleeping on a pool raft in a sleeping bag.

I surrendered all rights to beauty by this point. My friend I lived with was beautiful and everyone loved her. I think I was able to be friends with her because I had surrendered my rights to any of that. I slept on her floor the whole last quarter of school.

Now I was going to eat healthy. I couldn't eat the dorm food because that was my problem—that's why I couldn't abstain. I couldn't get the idea of no eating in between planned meals. I thought it had to be a strict food plan or nothing and those O.A. people were copping out.

I stayed crazy. I was really ashamed. I didn't tell anybody I went to O.A. I would sneak out. I knew a girl at school and I found out that she was in O.A.—we started going to meetings together. It was a major turning point because I realized that it was OK. Somehow it made it less horrible that I had an eating disorder. She was recovering, she had about a year of abstinence and she was a "moderate mealer." It was a turning point but I wasn't able to stay abstinent.

I came home for the summer and had a horrible summer with my boyfriend. I remember visiting him during that school year and he took me in and out of the back door of his dorm. He was completely ashamed of me. Part of it was probably because I was intruding on his life there, but I know he was ashamed of me.

I really hated him because he abandoned me. He just withdrew all emotional support. I'd try to talk about it with him and he'd shut off. I don't think he ever knew I had a problem with food or anything.

The following September, I finally started letting it be *enough* to have three meals a day, nothing in between. I hadn't been able to bear the idea of God, but during that summer I was kind of "acting as if." It was a real slow process to arrive at a concept of a Higher Power. By September though, I was able to make the surrender to a power greater than myself.

Even though I didn't have continuous abstinence during the summer, I had a will to live, a will to try. I came back to school a lot stronger.

After trying to follow a food plan all summer, I was easily at a point where I could do three meals a day with nothing in between. It was a major revelation that it was enough to do that. I started doing that and somehow I didn't have the health stuff intertwined anymore. I cared about the weight, but it was secondary to stopping the compulsive overeating.

Now I had peers. It was OK to be honest with a couple of different people about being in the program. Not everyone, just two people. I had a little less shame about it. I realized that I had nothing without abstinence. I was getting rid of the shame.

I remember in the first couple of days, before school started, I said to my O.A. friend, "I really need a meeting, let's go to a meeting." But then my roommate wanted me to drive her somewhere so I said OK. My friend confronted me and said, "You need to take care of yourself." I went to the meeting and let my roommate find another ride. I started being willing to brave somebody not being happy with the way I was changing. When you know it's a disease, it's easier to be honest. I didn't have to lie as much about things.

If I could recommend anything to somebody reading this, I'd say to get clear on the concept that it's a disease because that gets rid of a lot of "stinking thinking." It gets rid of a lot of the moral judgment and shame. I was able to be a lot more honest when I realized it wasn't something to do with my worth or my value as a person. Next, develop a concept of a power greater than yourself. That was so hard for me, but it didn't work for me without it. A commitment to self—there's nothing more important.

Get a bottom line for your abstinence—one you can live with continually. Mine's no eating in between planned meals. And get the whole health thing separated. I was so crazy about health and nutrition and weight. Get those separated somehow. I was lucky enough at that point, to have that recognition—that it didn't have anything to do with eating sugar or weight or whatever, it was just enough to stop the insanity of eating. I made a commitment to myself that this was the important thing in my life, even if I had to drop out of school. Abstain, no matter what. A life or death situation that I couldn't mess around with. I remember my mom saying, "Even if you have to sleep between breakfast, lunch and dinner, if nothing else, abstain.

I think some of the clarity I've gotten, like separating the health issues, and realizing what part of me is using the disease—how I used my eating disorder in my life to function—has brought me enough sanity and awareness that I never again have to be that person huddled in the bathroom stall.

THE WAY OUT

Steven M.

[Steven is 38 years old and has been abstinent from compulsive overeating for almost three years. He is a successful hairdresser who has done shows from New York to San Francisco. Steven remembers being teased about the way he ate as a child.]

I was about six years old when it was pointed out to me that the things I ate were real unusual, like a sandwich of grilled peanut butter and baloney and cheese all together. I'd fix it myself and put it in the broiler and broil it. I was kind of jokingly teased by my family. Like "Where did you learn to eat like that?" I know that when that attention would get focused on me it was highly uncomfortable.

At around eight or so, I started taking the little slivers off the cake and that kind of stuff to hide what I was doing. Like fluffing up the potato chip bag. Then I wouldn't have to listen to "Oh, you're eating again" or "Why are you eating that?" That's when I started getting up at night and going to the refrigerator. All these memories have become more vivid in recovery.

By the time I was eight or ten, I just knew that there was something the matter with me and that I wasn't supposed to be fat but I was. I mean, I was huge. I was in the fourth grade and there was only one kid in the sixth grade that was bigger than me. I was not only big in stature, but I was wide. I was a real big kid and people moved away from me when I walked down the halls. I felt safe. Nobody tried to beat me up. If anyone did call me a name, they ran. So there was a feeling of power and of being in control of that environment.

I usually had a least one friend and I had a brother I played with. So I wasn't totally alone but I can remember times of feeling like I was.

My mom put me on a diet by the time I was ten. My mom taught me to control my food. She put me on a severe diet, like salads and cottage cheese. I would lose a little bit of weight and then I don't know if they forgot about it or what. I was probably sneaking food for sure. I can remember that by the time I was in junior high I was putting myself on my own diets.

It was always a restrictive diet. It was the same food that was around the house, just less of it. My mother taught me a starch issue. I still think starch is just for clothes. Breads and potatoes and stuff like that; what she was always cutting back on was the carbohydrates. When I look back on it, that's probably one of the reasons why I was hungry all the time when I was a little kid. I was out burning it off and I didn't have anything to burn. I can remember times of not having any carbohydrates at all unless it was a glass of milk. It would only be meat and vegetables.

I don't think I ever really took all the weight off. I stayed big but I just wasn't as big. Or at least, my mind said that. I was 165 pounds in the sixth grade—that's big! I can remember pretty much staying that way all the way through junior high school.

[When Steven became a teenager and aware of girls, wanting to be thin became a very strong force. He began to get amphetamines from school buddies.]

I never got diet pills from a doctor. They were all street drugs. Except when we'd go to Mexico. I'd get prescription drugs there. You could go down there and get 1,000 pills for $25.00 back then. That's what everyone I knew in high school did on weekends. I also used LSD. I would not eat sometimes for four days.

I dropped out of school by the time I was 15. Remember "Turn on, tune in and drop out?" Well, I did it right in that order. I had developed antisocial attitudes. By then I was starting to be a hippie and have long hair and that was not acceptable at school. I was wearing beads and stuff. I guess I successfully ditched school for six months before I got caught. I intercepted all the letters from the school. I even forged signatures and sent them back. I truly thought that my father wouldn't find out.

When he did find out, I basically blackmailed my father. He said "Go back to school," and I said "No." I don't know how the system is now, but at that time your child was put into the California Youth Authority and they charged you a certain amount of money a day and I knew my father couldn't afford it. So I won out.

[Just before Steven's 16th birthday, his mother had a stroke and has been in the hospital ever since, for 22 years.]

After my mom's stroke, confrontations between my father and I grew. He basically left. He paid the rent and once in a while he would drop groceries off, if we were lucky. He was getting deeper and deeper into his alcoholism. I was taking care of everything by the time I was 17. I began dealing drugs. In fact, I got my own place with my brother. We just left.

I did have periodic attempts at trying to do certain types of work, but I would save enough money to get a kilo or something and then start dealing again and quit the job. You know the story, I felt I was never paid as much as I was worth and they should've made me foreman. As I got a little bit older I got construction jobs, but I always went back to dealing drugs because then I didn't want to deal with an authority figure.

[At about 25 years of age, Steven enrolled in beauty school.]

When I went to beauty school, I weighed 135. I starved myself to that weight with drugs and I still thought I was fat. In a way, I'm sure my industry fed my eating disorder. The beauty industry is a pretty unhealthy society. The fashion magazines have all kinds of unhealthy signals going out about body image and "looks" and things like that. I went from being a hippie with sandals and with my hair to my waist, right into this industry. I caught on real quick. It was about the looks. If you were thin enough and you looked good enough, you were going to make money in the business. I was real thin when I started out. It was one of the few times in my life when people were telling me I should put weight **on**.

I wasn't doing speed anymore or any psychedelics. I quit taking them because I was worried about my mental health. Not that I'd ever had a problem, but I was aware that if I kept taking LSD, something was going to happen.

I guess when I went to school I had something I wanted to do. I had to focus my energy, which I hadn't done in a long time. So I pretty much stayed away from most drugs for about three years. My weight slowly started creeping back up. I started to diet and crash diet to try to control my weight gain. That's when I started getting into cocaine. From the time I was about 27 to 34 years old, cocaine and starvation were my answer to controlling my weight.

In the beginning everything seemed just fine. My work was picking up. I wasn't doing a lot of heavy dealing at that time. I'd get a quarter of an ounce or so and sell it to pay for what I was using.

I stayed pretty much around 160 to 165 pounds and had girl-friends. I thought I was having the time of my life. I was partying, I had friends and looked good. I knew as long as I kept thin and I had money, I would have friends and lovers and be happy.

What started happening after awhile is the cocaine changed—the way it acted on me changed. It no longer suppressed my eating unless I did a quarter of an ounce in the morning. Instead of getting me excited and hyped, it calmed and mellowed me out. It was like ritalin for a hyperactive child. I was doing a half an ounce of cocaine a day and I was creeping up toward 200 pounds which seemed real unusual. Later, a doctor told me that it's not really uncommon for that to happen.

Now I was doing cocaine just to get out the door. I was doing it to go to the bathroom. I was doing it to put my clothes on. How you can get like that and not be aware of it, still escapes me.

I remember one incident toward to end of my using. I went on a nine-day drug and drinking binge. I didn't eat or sleep. I went through five ounces of cocaine and about $1500 on drinking. Then I crashed out for two days. I remember getting up and getting on the scale and getting really mad because I'd gained weight! I was furious! I'd gained about five pounds. I weighed between 190 and 200 pounds. I eventually got up to over 225.

I began having heart palpitations. I'd be doing cocaine and my heart would stop beating. I was gasping for air. I wasn't fun to be around anymore. People weren't coming home and partying with me after hours.

One time, I did a gram in just one line. I felt my heart pounding and then it stopped and I just fell over. I felt a real peace that I hadn't felt in a long, long time. I knew I was dying. I got tunnel vision where everything just faded out. I saw a white glowing light and then I got the incredible pain in my chest and my heart started beating again. I got dizzy and I crawled into the bathroom and tried to throw up in the toilet. I asked God why He didn't take me.

After that, I tried cleaning up because I knew I was killing myself.

[While Steven was trying to get off of cocaine, he met and got involved with a new woman.]

My new girlfriend was thin and little, probably anorexic. Her only desire in life was to be a nurse and now she found someone to take care of. Within a few weeks after I started seeing her, she moved in and the next thing I knew I was engaged for the first time in my life.

I was about $10,000 in debt when I stopped snorting cocaine. Within about six weeks of just dealing, it was paid off. I was saving money and I thought I was on top of the world. But I started to put weight back on, so I was back at trying to control my food again. I don't know if that's what caused me to start using the drugs again or not. But I began by licking the cocaine off my fingers when I would be packaging it up to sell. I was drinking rum and coke at the time and I started putting some in my drink. I got back into doing it that way. I was doing it like that for about two or three months. Nobody knew about it.

Pretty soon we were both using again and my girlfriend got down to about 85 pounds. I hadn't really noticed that she'd gotten that thin. She was maybe doing a gram or so a day. Unbeknownst to me, she began calling a cocaine hotline. If I had been on the other end of the phone, I would have been telling her to leave me too. We ended up breaking up.

The break up ripped me apart. I started doing a lot more drugs and drinking and partying, going out to the bars and chasing women around, trying to forget the pain and not feel it.

My career and my dealing started getting screwed up. I started losing money. What had been a promising career heading toward being a salon owner was gone. My drug connection had gotten so far in debt to the people he was doing business with that they cut him off. I had stopped doing business with other people, so then I was cut off too.

I quit doing drugs then, as far as I can remember. The withdraw-als were the most painful thing I've ever felt in my life. I felt like a malaria victim; I'd get the chills and the shakes. Somehow I was managing to get to work. I would drag myself. They didn't fire me. They would cancel my appointments for me and reschedule them and I'd crawl into the back office and lie down and shake.

After about two months, I started going to Cocaine Anonymous meetings. I kept going to meetings for a month before I quit drinking. I didn't hear that alcohol was a drug. About eight or nine months into my recovery from drugs and alcohol, I started being exposed to people from Overeaters Anonymous. I remember making jokes about it. I know now that was my way of denying my own problem.

Right after my one-year birthday in C.A. and A.A., I got sick and I hadn't been that sick in a long time. I had the chills and sweats and felt like the withdrawals all over again. I went to the refrigerator just like I used to go to the mirror and do the cocaine. The refrigerator was starting to look like a mirror.

One night, I had bought some cookies. I was hiding them all around the living room. Eight or nine over here, behind something where no one could see them and I could sneak them. And there wasn't anyone home. That bothered me. I moved them out of the hiding spot, but then I'd move them back. Then I hid them way back up in the cupboard. Then I ate the whole bag.

At that time, I weighed more than I'd ever weighed before in my life. I quit stepping on the scale when it hit 230. I was numb or I was frantic. When I was hiding those cookies, I knew something was wrong. You only hide drugs. Why am I hiding the cookies? I was so ashamed.

I just remember that fear of knowing something was the matter. I knew if I didn't do something, I was going to get stoned or drunk or both. I knew I was on the edge. So I called up the one person I could trust, a woman in A.A. who was also in O.A. I don't even remember now what she said to me, but I felt OK when we were done talking. I found out something was the matter with me and I wasn't bad, you know? It was a few days later that I went to an O.A. meeting.

The O.A. meetings were real confusing. Nothing made sense. I didn't want to be there and I was real angry so I didn't hear a lot. When I'm angry I don't hear very much. I don't get angry hardly any more.

I kept going to O.A. meetings. I'd hear someone share their story and I didn't relate to it yet. I knew I belonged there but I didn't understand why. I mean, I was an addict. It had just been a few months before that I admitted I was an alcoholic. My denial was real, real deep. I wanted to just be an addict and not have to hassle the rest.

I think where I started hearing something was at a meeting that had a lot of cross-addicted people attending it. I'd hear people talking and I knew they knew what I was feeling. They were alcoholics with eating disorders. I could relate to them. I trusted them.

In the beginning, I just abstained and went to meetings. All I knew was it felt like a diet. I was eating four times a day. I had three meals a day and I had a piece of fruit at night before I went to bed. What I got told was "don't eat in between meals." It was strongly suggested that I have only three, but I understood it was OK if I didn't. I continued on that way for probably for the first six to nine months. It was just control. I faked it until I started getting a concept of what it was all about.

What I got was, it didn't have to be like it had been all my life. There was a feeling of freedom from what my body looked like and from food making me OK. Somehow, that feeling of freedom was more important than the feeling that I didn't have to drink and use drugs any more. That feeling still is very, very important to me.

It was like this was the core, and the other shit was to cover this up. That's what made it really hard in the beginning. I knew that the drugs, the booze, were a symptom of something else. And then I came to believe that the way I ate and controlled my food was a symptom of something else too.

I was told to have trust and faith in God and just don't eat in between planned meals, no matter what, and wait for the miracle to happen. I listened to someone else for a change. I became vulnerable and I revealed who I was in front of a group of people, like I never had before in my life. I shared the best I could about what it was like and what happened to me and what I was becoming. I did not eat in between planned meals no matter what—no matter how sick I got, no matter how rejected I felt—all the feelings I'd eaten over before. I had to feel them this time.

If I hadn't found O.A., I don't know where I'd be today. I might be stoned or I'd be fat and sober and very unhappy because I had a lot of anger.

The quality of my life today has increased beyond anything I could have imagined because of O.A. It's a freedom I've never known before, not only from the food, but from a life style that I was so entrapped in, that I thought there was no way out. Overeaters Anonymous showed me the way out.

FULL RECOVERY, FULL LIFE

Teri K.

[Teri is 33 years old and has over four years of abstinence. She is a licensed Shiatsu therapist and a avid runner. Teri is a full-time student in her junior year at the local state university. It was in her teens that she first recalls an eating problem.]

My girlfriends and I, at about age 14, would smoke pot and then we'd have the munchies. We'd eat everything in the kitchen that we could find. It didn't matter whose house we were at. Nobody thought anything about it. But after awhile, I started staying home and isolating and not doing any drugs and just eating. I'd cry, I felt really afraid and I was really lonely.

I remember being terrified of men, or boys, at 14 and 15. When I was about 16, I had a boyfriend, but I didn't know how to talk to him. I felt like some kind of abnormal reject. I had horrible self-worth, terrible fears. I always felt like I didn't fit in. I stayed home. It was very comforting, but I knew it was abnormal. I was feeling really isolated.

I started doing diets. I probably weighed about 118, or 120 at the most, when I went on my first diet. I think I was trying to control my *weight*, I don't know, maybe I was trying to control my *eating*. I knew the minute I stopped dieting I'd start eating again, so I'm not sure.

I think I got the different diets from my girlfriends or books. I remember the Stillman diet, I remember the grapefruit diet. When my weight got to about 130 pounds, I went to a doctor and he gave me a prescription for diet pills. The prescription was renewable three times, after that he wouldn't renew it and he wouldn't write me another one either. I used the diet pills and didn't eat at all—that's how I did the "diet."

The summer before my senior year of high school, I stayed at my cousin's house and watched her kids. I ate the whole time. I realized there was something wrong with me. I kept looking in the mirror after I ate to see if my body was expanding. I already knew there was something wrong with the way I ate. My family was already hiding food from me.

I remember I found the ad for Overeaters Anonymous in the local Pennysaver. I saw it right before I left. I thought about it while I was taking care of my cousin's kids. I knew that probably nobody, even if they weighed 300 pounds, ate like I was eating. I thought I was abnormal.

When I got back from my cousin's, I looked for that ad. I remember finding it and looking at the ad, saying, "I wonder if they would think I was weird," you know, going in there when I only weighed about 125. I wondered if you have to be really heavy to go to this thing.

I dragged a girlfriend to my first meeting at the end of August. I identified immediately. They were all a lot heavier than me, except this one woman who walked in late. She was really thin and she looked really together. I wanted her to be my sponsor.

I remember everybody being accepting. There was not another person my age there—I was 17. I scooped up all this literature and went home and started reading it. All I remember is something about food plans. I don't remember much of anything else—just talking about the eating and then talking about the food plan. I took one home. It seemed like a diet but they called it a food plan. That was fine, I was used to doing that kind of stuff.

I remember feeling like I just didn't seem to be ready to stop. I realized that there were people who came to O.A. and were ready to stop.

I knew there was a real difference between people who were abstaining and people who were bingeing—me. I wanted what they had, but I didn't want to have to stop compulsively overeating.

I would get tough sponsors, then I would get easy sponsors. I kept bouncing back to my same old sponsor, the one that walked in that first night. Finally, one time, I went up to her and asked for a few minutes to talk to her. I told her I'd just broken my abstinence, again. She just took me by the shoulders and looked at me and said, "Teri, I just want to shake you. It's so painful watching you do this. You go and you quit your job and you break your abstinence and then you come to me and you ask me for some advice. You ask me if you did the right thing quitting your job, you tell me you broke your abstinence. You never call *before* you do any of that. You never call and ask for help before you eat. You never call before you quit your job. I just don't know what to do with you anymore."

This was a turning point for me. I felt like, oh, my God, I might actually drive myself out of O.A. Maybe O.A. people would really get sick of listening to me. Maybe I will not have this place to come to if I keep doing this. I was afraid that maybe O.A. wouldn't work for me and I would just alienate everyone around me and I knew that I would just die. Within the next month I started abstaining.

After I started abstaining, I felt part of the recovering group. But even after three months of abstinence, I remember feeling like that if things got bad enough, it was OK to binge. I still had this "hole card." About that time, I heard an A.A. speaker say that abstinence should be like sobriety— that you don't eat no matter what. I remember thinking, "OK, I've got to abstain, no matter what." And that feeling stayed with me until I started getting into relapse eight and a half years later. I know some kind of surrender took place.

I moved to Hawaii after I'd been abstinent about two and a half years. I was 22 years old. I met a man in A.A. through some friends. We started living together very quickly and then we got married. I thought it would be this perfect, beautiful little program marriage. We had a lot of things in common, a lot of common interests, the same kind of feeling about the program. He was probably the most supportive person to my O.A. program—who didn't have an eating disorder—that I've ever met. A clean and sober person who regarded it as important as sobriety and he respected my commitment to my recovery.

I had started running when I had about three months of abstinence. I call it my "fun runner" stage. I think I got this feeling like, "Wow, my body works!" The summer after we were married, I started getting into aerobic dancing. Exercise was still fun and it was a wonder to feel my body and play. We rode bikes too—it was all play.

When it turned serious, I must've been 24 or 25. I started training for races. You have to do these workouts. For the next four years it got real serious.

Running started to seem like part of my abstinence. Like I had to run, I had to do certain things in the day—all these things became abstinence. I really got abstinence, health and nutrition totally confused. Healthy living and abstinence got real mixed up. During that time, I'd go through a cycle where I'd be more obsessed with food and then I'd be less obsessed with food.

I became interested in running in a 10K. To train, I upped my miles to that distance, six miles. Little by little I increased my miles. I'd do a long run of four or five miles. I remember when I did my first six-mile run and how exciting that was.

Pretty soon I'd do six miles maybe twice a week and the rest of the time maybe two or three miles. From six miles, I went up to eight miles and then about ten miles. After my husband ran the Honolulu Marathon, I decided I wanted to train to run a marathon. I was running five or six days a week now. It went from about ten miles a week to about 25 and then, when I was training for the marathon, it got up to about 40 miles a week. I probably had one 50 mile week. It seemed like most people ran a lot more to train for a marathon, 50-60 miles a week, regularly.

The first marathon I trained for, I started eating to accommodate for—I was getting really thin, overly thin. It was hard for me to increase my portions and to eat more calorie dense carbohydrates. It took someone sitting me down and saying, "You have got to eat for a runner—you have got to change the way you eat. I don't care what they say in O.A., we've got to do something here or you're going to waste away." So I upped my carbohydrates, I ate three good-sized meals a day, mostly centered around complex carbohydrates. I was a vegetarian so they were all complex carbohydrates.

[As Teri's weight dropped almost ten pounds, she became more and more obsessed.]

I was really caught up in being thin—very caught up in my body image. My body image was screwed up the whole time I was abstinent—I never talked about it and I never heard it talked about. On a daily basis, I'd look in the mirror and see how much my stomach stuck out. I weighed about 105. I just never saw myself realistically. I might at times, but everything depended on how flat my stomach was. I remember my husband saying to me, "You know Teri, you seem to have a good program, you seem to have a lot more freedom with abstinence than most people I know, but the way you are around your body is sort of sick, sort of weird." I remember he said it in a real gentle way, but it sure was accurate.

I don't remember other feelings, I only remember the feeling of needing to control. I remember the scariest feeling was being out-of-control. Not usually with eating, that didn't come until my relapse, but with my surroundings—my work, my running, my marriage.

I was into long-distance running. I was into my profession, Shiatsu therapy. I remember feeling that I've got to keep up all this stuff. I've got to keep up my profession, I've got to be really good. I've got to keep up in my running. I've got to train for marathons because that made me what I was. I didn't talk in meetings about how really desperate I felt sometimes, especially about my relationship with my husband. I felt like I couldn't live with this man and I couldn't live without him.

There was a tremendous amount of verbal abuse, fighting all the time. Intellectual abuse mostly, any time I would try and detach from him at all. We finally separated when I was 28. Although I remember feeling a lot of relief not being around his energy, we got back together because I felt like I hadn't stopped loving this man and I couldn't live without him.

Back together, I just worked even harder at my profession. I felt like I had to do these things to make me OK. It's what validated me. Being married validated me. I wasn't anything alone.

We were together maybe only one month when I really knew that nothing had changed. I felt like my heart was just breaking. It was so awful—the realization that he hadn't changed. He had tried to convince me that he had changed and that he wasn't going to be clingy and abusive. I realized that he had really just done that to get me back. I hadn't changed either. I was right back into being clingy and dependent, with everything revolving around him instead of being my own person.

I was still abstaining. I wasn't having any relapse symptoms that I recognized at that time. I was working a lot and then I hurt my back. I couldn't move. I mean, there was a period of time when I just lay on the couch with a heating pad. I couldn't run. I couldn't do my work—I had to quit doing Shiatsu. I felt like my whole world was falling apart and I was nothing. I remember staying home and starting to add to my meals at lunch, like going to the refrigerator and getting a big scoop of peanut butter. That was after eating the meal in front of me. I knew it was starting to get bad.

Then I started stretching the meal by going back and getting more food for, maybe, the next hour after my lunch. I remember feeling guilty, thinking, "I can't tell anybody about this," and feeling scared. I finally told my husband, "I'm having some problems." He started coming home and saying, "Well, were you OK today?" and I'd lie to him. Neither one of us really talked honestly about what was happening.

. I was stretching meals beyond the limit and I was starting to go crazy because my weight was going up. One day, a few months later, I remember I went out after lunch. It was an hour after lunch and I was on my way to an O.A. meeting. I drove to a health food store and got this big goodie. After I ate it, I thought, "I broke my abstinence, I can't call that a meal." I flipped out. I went home and I told my husband—he flipped out too. We were both crying and going crazy and being hysterical.

I had had eight and a half years, I would've had nine years in three months. We decided not to tell. Somehow we rationalized it, "No, you really didn't break your abstinence, it was only an hour after an meal." It started getting worse. I'd eat a meal then I'd go to the movies and I'd eat another meal. It got crazy. I really would try to abstain. I never told anybody at the O.A. meetings, I had the longest period of abstinence on the islands—I knew I was going crazy.

I was terrified of letting go of my husband, I couldn't decide about the marriage and I couldn't abstain. I was desperate. During that relapse, the mental obsession with eating was so bad that I wanted to put a gun to head on a daily basis.

I heard of a recovery home for eating disorders. A place that just used the 12 Steps, non-clinical. They ate three moderate meals a day, didn't ban any foods and it was in the desert area around Los Angeles. I saw a brochure but I vacillated.

I finally called up the recovery home. I went for a screening. After talking to different people in the program, I decided to go in. I went and I was terrified. When I got there, I was three days abstinent. I walked in the door and it felt like I was done—I'll do whatever they want me to do, I don't care what it is, I'll do it, I don't care what they have me eat.

Hearing what they said, I knew in my heart it was recovery. I remember asking the director, "Are you sure I never have to go back out again? I'm a relapse person, I'm a retread. Are you sure this will last me the rest of my life?" She told me, I never have to compulsively overeat again. She said I could be abstinent the rest of my life, one day at a time.

I made a decision I would do whatever I needed to do to recover. I think when I got willing to abstain, no matter what, I had to find an abstinence I could live with a day at a time for the rest of my life. I had to find some kind of Higher Power and support. I didn't believe so much in God at that time. I felt abandoned by Him. I made a decision to work the Steps with a sponsor and a support group, as much as possible.

The director said to me, and I really believe that this is true, "The issues that you didn't deal with before—the ones that contributed to the relapse—have to do with codependency." Now, I also go to Codependents Anonymous too. I'm going to a therapist who's helping me deal with the codependency issues and she honors my commitment to my 12-Step programs. That's the way I need to deal with the codependency issues, really full on, head on. By doing that, I've found a lot of recovery in my relationships. It's ongoing. I've been able to have some reparation take place with my family too. It's a miracle.

[Teri went back to school after two years of abstinence and is a member of the track team, a long distance runner.]

Things are different now. My running, my healthy eating, they only add to my life. They don't define me. Sometimes there's a fine line for me between training and getting compulsive again, but I'm willing to be honest about it and talk about it. What I think I have learned is, how running can **add** to my life, not be my whole life. Today it's OK for running to be in my life. For awhile, I thought it wasn't OK to run again.

I think that being abstinent and recovering gives us life back. I don't feel like there's any limit to what I can do today. I don't have to live like a handicapped person. I know I have things to learn and I've got a lot of growing to do but I don't have to worry about the things I worried about in my disease. I don't have to be controlled by it any more.

FROM DIETING MADNESS TO DISEASE RECOVERY

Jean M.

[Jean M. is a 61-year-old woman with almost four years of abstinence from compulsive overeating. She has been active in sports all her life. Jean doesn't recall any concern about her weight or eating during her childhood.]

I lived in a little town in the mid-west and I'd ride my bicycle down to the store every night in the summer and get a pint of ice cream. At the time I don't think I thought much about it. It seemed a normal thing to do. During high school, one of the things I used to do was open a can of peas and have that for breakfast—the whole can. These are things I thought of later, now it seems like that wasn't normal—not how most people would have eaten.

[Jean was a professional dancer in her teens. She married and had her first child at 19 years of age, at which time she began to gain weight.]

I felt that I had gained weight because of the pregnancy and that I'd probably lose it. But from then on it was like a roller coaster—up and down with my weight continually. I had four children, all of them two and one half years apart. With my fourth child, I'd gained something like 30 or 40 pounds during my pregnancy and I kept that weight on longer.

I remember my husband buying me a size 18 dress. I was very unhappy about that, when he bought the dress. I brought it back and I think I exchanged it. That wasn't the size I wore. I was maybe a size 16 at the height of 5'9". I think I was probably a 12 when I got married. It was a nice gesture. He was not being mean. He just felt I needed a new dress, but it really hurt.

I got diets from magazines. I'd always go on the latest "fad" diet. They would all work for awhile. Something new seemed to help me each time, but it wouldn't last.

My husband was a psychiatrist and after the last child was born we came to California to live. After about five years of on-and-off dieting, one of my husband's physician friends gave me diet pills. Later the pharmacist would give them to me. I didn't abuse them. As a matter of fact, I wouldn't say I took them abusively in any way. I took one a day and sometimes I even cut down and didn't take it because they made me so nervous. Sometimes I'd take the capsules apart and just take part of it instead of the whole thing. I also remember going down to Mexico to a "fat farm" resort for a week. I don't recall what my weight was. I would fluctuate a lot.

Between the ages of 30 and 40, my weight just kind of went up and down. It was still the same 15-20 pounds—I didn't get into a higher bracket. This was when I used the diet pills and I was drinking then. More than once or twice a year I'd gain and lose. Sometimes I'd keep using the diet pills to keep it off.

I just thought that everyone had to go on a diet. It was something that most people did. A lot of people had problems with weight and so did I. I would take the diet pills and then I'd get real nervous, so I'd drink for a couple of days. I would get so horribly sick when I drank that I couldn't lift my head off the pillow so I'd stay in bed. Then I'd start eating for a couple of days. Then I might go back and start taking the diet pills until I got too nervous and uptight again. Then it would be the same thing all over again. Sometimes I'd stick to the diet for maybe a week or two without drinking. I was a periodic drinker.

I had gotten one drunk driving arrest toward the end of my marriage. I got divorced in September of 1970 and I joined Alcoholics

Anonymous in February of 1971. Toward the end of 1971, a few of us in A.A. tried Overeaters Anonymous to deal with our weight problems.

My first A.A. sponsor went with us to O.A. She didn't like it so we had our *own* meeting at her house. We didn't really run it like an O.A. meeting—we'd all weigh in. I don't remember, but I think we met at her house once a week. That went on for six to eight months. Then two of us went to get those weight-loss shots. She lost her weight but I wasn't successful. I went back to O.A. at that point.

I managed to keep some of my weight off for quite a while. I was having a love affair and did pretty well for a couple of years, not feeling there was anything seriously wrong with me. I wasn't abusing food much at that time, I don't know why. I guess because my life was going pretty well. I was enjoying myself. I wasn't over-exercising.

Although my weight was up there when I met him, I began to lose weight. I remember I couldn't go to bed with him at first but then I lost weight. He made the comment that he didn't like me that thin. He said later that he liked me a little bit heavier. I was back down to a 14.

At the time the love affair ended, I had been a little heavier but then I lost some weight. During this time I had the longest abstinence I'd ever had. I was very active in O.A.

I went crazy when I found out he started living with somebody else. It was a black-out period for me. I went from 165 pounds to 240 pounds. I wasn't talking to anybody. I hadn't told any of my friends I was having this affair with him. I did keep going to A.A. meetings but I don't remember continuing with O.A.

I think I always thought it was a weight problem, not an eating problem. Just eating too much and not exercising enough. I didn't understand it was a disease. I think at some points in there I would've had longer periods of abstinence if I had the understanding that I do today, that you eat three meals a day with nothing in between. Because many times I would eat a piece of cake,—just one piece of cake *with* my meal—and think I broke my abstinence.

I got so miserable I couldn't stand it anymore. I went to therapy, individual and groups and I went to A.A. meetings. I was on antidepressants during that time. I always hung around A.A. because I was successful there.

I went to therapy for a long time and I didn't seem to get any help. All we talked about was my eating and weight. I think the therapist had an eating disorder too. We just talked in terms of weight.

I just hated myself because I was so heavy. I'd broken up the relationship and that wasn't what I wanted. I wasn't honest with him. I didn't tell him that I wanted to live with him. I just walked away from the relationship and I didn't communicate with him at all on anything. I felt angry with myself because I hadn't shared that. I didn't communicate with people about what was going on with me. Some of my best friends didn't even know—I wouldn't share with them. I was staying away from my sponsor.

I'd go to O.A. meetings and think, God why can't I get this, there's something wrong with me. Why can't I get this? I was suicidal.

My best friend talked to my daughter, who is sober in A.A., and they planned an intervention. From the intervention I learned they cared and also that I was in trouble, which I already knew. I knew that I was in trouble but I still didn't think of it as a disease. I thought I was just overweight and I could lose weight again as I always had in the past with a diet. I thought that I was just sick emotionally and psychologically.

I wouldn't go into the hospital treatment program because of the money. I wouldn't part with the $18,000 and I didn't have insurance. I heard about a recovery home that used the 12 Steps of Overeaters Anonymous. I called to get an interview. After a few weeks I finally got in.

In the beginning, I used to have a thought, Oh my God, here I am at a recovery home and I hear about people out there breaking their abstinence and what if the same thing happens to me. Then I thought, that doesn't have to be you, Jean. That's what it's been in the past and now I know it's a disease. That's one thing I realized—*from a diet to a disease.*

What I finally got was that the power to abstain comes from our Higher Power and it comes from within and that there isn't somebody out there that's gonna do it and you have to do it yourself and it's tough. I did have a Higher Power, for the moment, so I could begin to like myself again. I got trust in myself again. That's another thing I got. I remember leaving the recovery home after four months and saying "I'm trustworthy," and I hadn't believed that for years.

Going to the recovery home was very important to me because I'd been around for so long. By going to the recovery home I was able to get my self-respect back.

Something I still work on is sharing with people and not isolating. That's very important for me. I also learned to be honest with people and to not be afraid. I definitely remember leaving there thinking I can trust myself.

By then I was able to surrender and know that this was a disease and I wasn't a bad person. I learned this is not a diet. This is a disease. You can eat three meals a day. Now I realize that we have grey areas sometimes and particularly in the beginning of recovery. But we just eat three meals a day anyway.

And I definitely need to keep using the tools, particularly sharing with somebody, sharing everything whether you think it's important or not. You need to have a relationship with somebody where you're talking all the time. I think sharing your experience, strength and hope regardless of what it is, high or low or whatever, sharing it continually, is important.

I didn't get into the Steps in the beginning when I went to A.A. and I think that was a mistake. I didn't have sponsors who got into the Steps. I think it's definitely important that we be told you must work the 12 Steps.

I've been really happy with my recovery now. I'm really proud of myself and how I've improved. It's all about growth for me.

RECOVERY FROM SELF-WILL RUN RIOT

Jerry J.

[Jerry is a 41-year-old computer technician who's been in the Navy for 16 years. A handsome black man with over two years of abstinence, awareness of a problem only came with weight gains as an adult.]

When I was about 25, I was a civilian working for our government in Vietnam. In Vietnam, being fat is a sign of prestige. So when I started putting on weight, it was OK, tailor-made suits cost like $40.00. The weight didn't matter, it was no big issue.

No one judged my weight but me. It wasn't really so much the weight as I felt *out-of-control*. I would drink so I wouldn't eat and then I would eat so I wouldn't drink. The feelings of being out-of-control with my drinking or my eating were what I remember being uncomfortable with. Other times though, I remember I would eat more so I could drink more.

I stayed in Vietnam two and a half years. I got married just before I left Vietnam. I came to Oakland with a Vietnamese wife. I probably got married for all the wrong reasons. She treated me like a god. I knew that I wouldn't be able to find another woman like that. It wasn't so much a thing of love as it was my need to be taken care of, and that's what she did, she took very good care of me. When I would drink and I had trouble getting up in the morning, she'd make sure I got up and went to work.

We lived together for two years before we got married. When I look at it now, I was just a man-child and she did an excellent job of taking care of this grown man-child.

In the beginning she didn't want to come to America because she had a lot of fear that maybe I would desert her once I brought her here. What I mean by that is, I was always out running the streets chasing after other women and at times, I would spend the rent money instead of paying it.

Her family was real glad that she got married. She had a son and I adopted him. They were all glad she was finally married because that made her "legitimate." Her mother told her—I loved her mother for this—if there's anything wrong with the marriage, it's your duty to fix it. My family liked her because it settled me down. My family remembered me when I was in the height of my drinking, so my family was all for anything that would settle me down.

She did get Americanized, but I think a big part of it had to do with my drinking. When I was drinking there were times when I would knock her around. I remember she used to wear these big sunglasses because they would cover her black eyes. I remember one time I got arrested for "driving under the influence." I called her to bail me out, and she said "I didn't tell you to get behind the wheel and drive." Click. She got sick and tired of my behavior. When I stopped drinking, started getting better and I wasn't such a child to take care of, her energies were more directed to herself.

I decided to join the Navy. In order to get in the Navy, I had to lose weight. That began the focus on the weight. I just stopped eating until I was at the "right" weight, then I got in. That was my first attempt at weight loss—a fast. Once I got in the Navy, I didn't think they were going to mess with me over my weight, so I didn't care. I went back to eating the way I normally did.

I was stationed in Pensacola, Florida, and the Navy intervened on me—they put me in the weight-control program there. They used to weigh me twice a month. I'd always fast for three days before I got weighed-in and then I'd binge three days after I weighed in. That kept my weight kind of steady.

I've stayed on the Navy's weight-control program for 12 of the 16 years I've been in. Each command was a little different. Basically, there was a lot of dishonesty in the weigh-ins and it depended on whether I knew the guy who was weighing me in. If I knew the guy, he'd say he didn't want to put down that I had gained weight because the C.O. would rag on me, so he'd put me down as the same weight. It sounded good to me. The guy would weigh me in and falsify records that I weighed less.

When it came to advancement, though, I **had** to be a certain weight. The first time to be advanced, I had to lose 40 pounds. I just stopped eating for 30 days and the weight came off. Then I went back to eating "normally." About three and a half years later I had to lose 55 pounds to be advanced again. I guess my body's smarter than me because this time I couldn't fast for 30 days. So I fasted for three weeks, ate for three days, then fasted for another three weeks. I still had a pound and a half to go. I decided I would seek some outside help.

I went and asked some of my Navy buddies what they did. One guy told me to take a whole bottle of Milk of Magnesia and that would clean my system out. I thought that should be good for a pound and a half. So I did that, but it was only good for three-quarters of a pound. I went and asked another Navy buddy what he did, and he said just go out and run until you can't run any further. I went out and ran about 15 miles. I put a dime in the phone, called my wife and asked her to come and pick me up—I couldn't get home. The next day I crawled up to the scale and I was at the medical weight to be advanced. A friend of mine gave me a five-pound box of chocolates, which I proceeded to reward myself with after the weigh-in. After all that agony I went through to get there!

My weight just went up after that. I had gotten to the point where I knew I just couldn't lose weight, they'd just have to kick me out or send me to treatment. Somebody had told me about a guy that used to weigh 100 pounds more than he did now. I talked to him and he said, "I went to N.A.R.C. Miramar." I said, "Yeah, that's Navy Alcohol Rehab."

[Jerry had been through the Navy treatment program for his alcoholism several years before and had been sober for about five years.]

He said they had an eating disorder section that he went through and now he eats anything he wants to in *moderation* and he's maintained a 100-pound weight loss for a year. I asked him how to get in. He said I need to get recommended by the counseling center. I got recommended for Level 3 treatment, which is in-patient for six weeks. That was April but I didn't get in until November of 1986.

In the Navy treatment program, they introduced me to O.A.'s 12 Steps and they bused us to O.A. meetings all around San Diego. After going through N.A.R.C., I had my first slip. I'd get about 60 days of abstinence and things would start working in my life and I'd be uncomfortable with it being calm and I'd eat again. I did that three times before I really looked and thought, "What do other people do in this program? Why isn't it working for me?" I watched and listened, and I heard people talk about getting a sponsor. I decided to get one. I asked about 40 guys to sponsor me, and everybody said no. I thought, "I'm screwed up now, I'll never get a sponsor."

The next week I went to a meeting and I asked the guy who led it to be my sponsor. For the next 30 days, he had me do reading and writing assignments. When the 60 days came around again and I got that same uncomfortable feeling, I called and told him. He said, **"You're just feeling a little serenity. It's OK, it'll pass, and no, you don't have to eat!"**

I kept abstaining. I was going to a lot of meetings. I wasn't willing to do my fourth step—the inventory of my past—yet because I knew instinctively that it meant that I would have to eventually make amends to myself and to other people. That meant I would have to quit doing certain behaviors—I would have to be faithful to my wife. I just wasn't sure.

It took me almost a year to do my fourth step. I knew it meant change. I hated change. I remember finally getting it done and sharing it with my sponsor. We met in a park. After I read it to him, he gave me a hug. I thought this is not the most macho thing I could be doing today. But the second thought was that I had just dumped all my garbage and I wanted to know in my heart that I was OK. When he gave me the hug, I felt OK so I just let it be.

He kept pushing me to continue working the Steps. I got through the sixth and the seventh step and then I got to the eighth step. I started making amends. I said to myself, "Well, I'll be on the ninth step the rest of my life." I talked to my sponsor about it and he said, "Make the amends you can and get on to the tenth step—start doing your daily inventory." I didn't like doing a daily inventory because it meant I had to be honest about my food, my family, my finances. I didn't want to be honest about those things. I would do it once a week, maybe twice a week, maybe every other week, whatever, but not daily.

My sponsor and I started growing apart. He broke his abstinence and left the program. I got a new sponsor and he started me over on the Steps. I did another fourth step.

What I was able to see in my second fourth step is a lot of stuff about sex, about things I stole in my life, about harm I intentionally did to other people. I felt the reason that much more came up was because God felt I was healthy enough to handle it this time.

A lot of things came up in this inventory about homosexuality. It was real hard for me to accept.

When I was 18 and I was at work, this one guy "dry humped" me. I felt so much shame about that. The biggest thing at the time was I didn't know I could tell him to stop. I didn't know how to stand up for myself and I didn't know I had a right to stand up.

Another memory was as a perpetrator on the kid next door. He was younger than me about a year. He was maybe 16 or 17. It started off real innocently. We would compare sizes to see who was bigger. It's like we sort of used each other. I can remember those times when he wouldn't do what I wanted him to do, I would have one of my drinking buddies go kick his ass.

The shame that came up around being sexually abusive and being sexually abused was overwhelming. It was more around the abusive behaviors. I didn't have warm or romantic feelings toward men—only shame for the way I treated them, for the way I treated me.

My sponsor told me I had to make amends to that younger "Jerry" who went through that abuse. He said I was probably still traumatized by it. I knew instinctively that I would probably never be able to make amends to the kid next door. But I knew at this time, I had to change my behaviors. I had to establish a sane and sound ideal around sex and where I was coming from with it. I spent more time reading the Alcoholics Anonymous big book, more time working on solutions.

I think what made it work—to continuously abstain—was to get a sponsor and to get a definition of abstinence that worked. In the beginning, what I did was I made my abstinence all-encompassing; if I went to a meeting, if I exercised, if I read some spiritual books, _then_ I was abstinent. In the beginning, I can remember those days when my eating was OK, but

I'd beat myself up because I didn't do the other things. What worked was getting a definition of abstinence that was just about my compulsive overeating.

In the beginning I followed the guidelines that I got from the Navy, which was three moderate meals a day. But as I progressed, I can remember on some days how that third meal got to be like a "wild card." I didn't always have time to eat three meals but I'd stick it in somewhere anyway. I used to hear people quote the <u>Overeaters Anonymous</u> book of "no eating in between planned meals." There was a recovery home in the area that would have brunch and dinner on weekends. I thought, "yeah, that works." There are days when I have brunch and dinner and I don't keep that third meal as a wild card. It was making me real insane to sit down real late, maybe after ten o'clock, and eat that third meal. A lot of things just started unfolding. People I was sponsoring started staying in recovery—getting long-term abstinence. It was showing me the program worked.

The thing that I'd want others to hear is that it's a disease and it's not a moral issue. That we're not good or bad because we can't control our eating or weight or body size. Another thing is to know as long as they keep coming back they get better. I've seen people in the program who have been coming around maybe ten years, but who only have three or four years of abstinence. It just shows me as long as I keep coming back I'll get better and there's hope. You don't have to do this alone, either. Don't waste any time in getting a sponsor and don't waste any time in getting your fourth step done. I see in my recovery today, my turning point was when I was willing to do my inventory. I had a lot more peace and calm once I did it.

The last thing I would share about my recovery is that I have found there are other 12-Step programs that help me. Be open-minded about them. I've gone to Alanon and CODA (Codependents Anonymous) and they've really helped me. Something I've been avoiding is therapy but I know it will probably help me. I'm just not there yet.

Once I was willing to not be so self-indulgent and say that maybe there's another way, my life got better. One more thing I want to say, something my very first sponsor taught me, to be gentle with myself. That's really what I needed and he really helped me to do it.

I THOUGHT I HAD TO BE OLD

Kathy R.

[Kathy's 25 years old and has over five years of abstinence. She's an attractive business executive who has a B.S. in accounting and is currently managing an accounting department. Kathy recalls the pain of being an overweight child.]

My first memories were when I was probably nine or ten years old. I remember even then having a relationship with food that I knew other people didn't have. I knew they didn't like it as much as I did. I would hide to eat it; I would eat in secret. I knew that I had a different thing with food than the other kids, but it was like my mom's relationship with food so it seemed somewhat normal at home.

I felt like there was something really wrong with my mom and me. It felt like we were *bad*. I was told that—that we were bad. My dad told me that. My brother told me that. My mom told me that. Everybody told me that I was bad if I ate.

My parents took me to the doctor when I was about nine. They said I had to lose weight. I don't really remember going, but after I got abstinent, I read my childhood medical records. Every month they would take me to the doctor and I would've gained two or three more pounds.

I didn't trade clothes with the other girls. My clothes were definitely bigger than theirs, that's how I know I carried more weight than normal. I can remember being teased really early as a kid, being called "fatty" when I was nine or ten. And it continued. I would get very, very angry when they would call me names or make remarks.

My dad was in the military and I went to school on the base until I was in ninth grade. I had a lot of friends and I did a lot of things with people. They were my friends and they were mean in a teasing kind of fun way. I had to be friends with people who teased me, because otherwise I would've been really, really alone.

I had been put a grade ahead; I skipped second grade. I was a bright little kid and it definitely influenced my self-esteem. I thought I was smarter and, therefore, better than they were. There was no in between. Either I was better or I was worse.

My dad had started going to A.A. when I was about eleven but he kept it a secret in the beginning. My mom started going to Overeaters Anonymous when I was a sophomore in high school—I was 14. She kept it a secret just like my dad did. My parents used to keep a lot of secrets from the children, but somehow we always found out about it.

We started going to Alateen when my dad had been sober for nine months. My mom kept O.A. a secret for, I guess, about six months. I remember finding out, I was really snoopy. I picked up the Alcoholics Anonymous book and she had crossed out all the words "alcohol" and had put "food." I thought it was kind of strange, but I knew it must be working for her because she seemed happier. She lost a lot of weight and had friends and was going places and doing things.

It seemed like it was an answer for her, but I felt like O.A. was for old people. I felt like I was too young. At that time, I really believed that once I got away from my mother and father and especially my brother, that my life would be fine, really fine. At home my brother would beat me up and my parents would not acknowledge that there was a problem. I used to think that my parents were really different from other people, like there was something wrong with them. I didn't feel like they understood me. I didn't feel like they wanted me. I didn't feel like they loved me. And

I didn't want to be like them.

We left the base in Spain when I got into high school. I was wearing size 16 pants when I was a sophomore in high school.

When I got a driver's license, I was happier. I knew I was leaving soon to go to college, away from home. But when I went to college, my weight just skyrocketed—I grew out of all my clothes real fast. The first semester of college, I gained at least 20 or 25 pounds.

I worked at McDonalds. It was really a fun place to work. I used to work the closing shift so if I was having a bad time, I would eat everything at night. I'd eat like a little bit of anything that was in the bin, french fries, a little bit of chocolate shake, massive quantities of diet soda. I'd go home and not be able to go to sleep for hours. I didn't know why.

At that point, I started reading books about nutrition to find out what was going on. My mom started telling me things like sugar is bad for you. She started teaching me about nutrition and trying to channel me toward controlling my weight with nutrition.

I can remember trying to go without eating at all. Then I'd end up just having some crackers in the afternoon, I'd end up getting really light-headed from not eating. I couldn't study.

I started taking the blame off of my family and putting it on me. Feeling like there must be something really wrong with me. I didn't understand. Why am I gaining weight? I felt like I was just eating pretty normally. I didn't binge, I didn't throw up—I never even heard of that. It didn't feel like I did anything excessively, except I had this problem with junk food and sweets.

At the end of my first year of college, I switched schools and moved back home with my mother and father. When we were apart, I realized that there were some things about them I really did like. Even though I didn't feel like they protected me, somehow it felt safe with them because they were familiar.

When I moved into the house, I took my mom's diet—it was an O.A. food plan—I stuck it up on the refrigerator and said, "I'm going to do this," and I did. That's the only time I remember sticking to a diet.

I had this concept that O.A. was a diet club. My dad used to call it mom's "get skinny club." That's what he called Weight Watcher's, that's what he called TOPS, and that's what he called O.A. I believed it was one more place that my mom went to lose weight. While I followed the food plan, I lost weight and leveled out in a bearable range again.

I started my third year of school. My weight kept going up and down and up and down within a 10-pound range. When I was about 19, it started to creep up again and I had no control. I'd just eat and I couldn't help it. I didn't understand it.

I never made friends at school. I always felt less-than. It really, really made me feel fat and ugly. That was a world I would never be able to belong to, but my grades were great. I felt like getting good grades was the only thing I could do right. I graduated from high school when I was 16 and I went to college. I had this long-range goal—I didn't want to be like my parents.

I had gotten involved in doing a lot of Alateen/Alanon service work. I was involved with people who seemed really happy all the time. I was supposed to be happy too because I was doing the same things they were, but I was miserable. One time I remember going to somebody's house to pick up this shipment of Alateen conference T-shirts and they had a scale in their bathroom. I stepped on it, when it got to 175 I jumped off because I got scared. My pants were getting tighter and tighter and I only had one pair—it was awful. I felt like if I stopped eating completely my body would still keep growing. Somehow I thought my body would get bigger and smaller based on my emotional health.

I had been going to Alanon since I was 18. There was a particular meeting that I went to and I started hearing a lot about Overeaters Anonymous. It used to make me really mad—I'd think "why are these weird people coming to my Alanon meeting? They should just go to their own meetings, and alcoholics too, they should just go to their own meetings and leave us alone."

There was a woman at my Alanon meeting who went to O.A. She asked me if I'd take her daughter to an Alateen meeting and I said, "I will if you'll take me to an O.A. meeting." I had no intention of saying that.

At that first O.A. meeting I heard "How it Works" read and other parts of the Alcoholics Anonymous book. I had known for a number of years that my father had stayed sober and was still sober. I figured if he could do that, then I could do this. I really got it that they were the exact same thing! If he could be so awful with his drinking and stay sober for eight years, then I could do this for a couple of years or a couple of months, or however long it would take to get all my weight off. That's really why I went—because my weight was at a point where I was going to kill myself.

The Steps and the program principles weren't new information, but the part about being able to turn over my eating and my food meant that now I was able to turn everything over to a Higher Power. It meant absorbing them into all areas of my life—my eating, my relationships with people, my work, my outlook on life. I had surrendered many different kinds of issues in the past, but it always felt like there was something missing. When I finally got it in my head that I could turn over my eating disorder to God, then I could surrender all of myself.

There was one woman at the meeting who was maybe 24 or 25 and she was abstinent and she talked about doing the same things the other older people did. She was one of the reasons I felt like it was OK to keep coming back. Nowadays there are a lot more young people in O.A. I think it's really important for young people to hear that, that you can arrest it at a young age.

I got abstinent when I was 20, so I was pretty young when I "got it," and I really believe I got it. It gave me a new outlook on life. I finally felt like I wasn't bad. I found out why I felt so different from everybody. After coming to O.A., it was like "Wow, a lot of people feel this way." I never knew that.

I WASN'T READY

Laura B.

[Laura is a vivacious 19 year old just beginning a career in the entertainment industry. She will celebrate four years of abstinence in November. She had no conscious awareness of an eating problem until she went into a recovery home for her drug and alcohol problem at the age of 15.]

I guess I chose people to be around me when I was younger who had eating disorders, so I wouldn't have to look at mine. I surrounded myself with people who had the compulsion to eat and were obsessed with food and weight. Even my friends who were thin. Now that I look back, they all had eating disorders. I recently found out one of them was vomiting, one of them was compulsively exercising, one of them, I guess, could just eat whatever quantities she wanted and not gain a pound, and one of them was overweight.

I remember I would go to school and not eat all day, come home and snack all night. I thought everyone did that because my friends were doing it too. I remember a few diets, but I thought everybody dieted. I thought my metabolism was different, because it appeared to me that people around me were eating more than me if not the same amounts, but I was heavier than they were.

I have memories of being uncomfortable with my body, I guess as young as eight or nine. I felt too fat, particularly in my stomach and my buns. My brother told me that, but mainly, it was my own awareness. The older I got, the more I dressed to hide my fat—my stomach and my thighs. I think I went between ten and probably twenty pounds overweight growing up.

I don't remember taking any specific drugs so I wouldn't eat, because when I smoked marijuana I would eat more. Everybody knew that when you smoked marijuana you got the munchies and that was why you were eating, because you were high and you had the munchies. That gave me permission, an excuse.

I started using speed but I didn't realize what it did until after I started using it. It made me not want to eat at all. The thought of food would nauseate me. That was exciting to me because I dropped a lot of weight. I dropped about ten pounds because I would go on two-week speed binges and not eat except maybe once or twice.

With the speed, the weight just came off and it stopped the desire to eat—I just didn't have any desire to eat. Looking back, I recognize that marijuana gave me permission to eat, and the speed eliminated the desire to eat.

When I got clean and sober, I was forced to look at my eating. They forced me to look at it as part of being in the recovery home. My mother told them I had an eating disorder—I was sent to O.A. Really, it felt like I was "sentenced" to O.A. and I hated it. The staff told me I had to eat three meals a day but I didn't—I didn't care. I wasn't hiding the fact that I wasn't eating three meals a day. When they confronted me, they said I either had to do it or I had to leave. They said that if I didn't arrest both diseases, I'd probably relapse. It was important to me to *get* and *stay* sober, so I did it.

The only way that I could come to any peace was to look at it and get honest about it. There was a little bit of freedom, in the beginning, but I didn't appreciate it. I was very pissed off that this was happening.

I didn't want to admit it until I was forced to. Maybe if I was never forced to, I might not have faced it yet. I never really felt I hit a bottom with my eating. I knew that my life was going bankrupt but I thought it was the drugs. If I had the choice sitting there in front of me— drugs, alcohol or food—I would take the drugs, first thing. Eating never put me into oblivion. It just made me more remorseful. It didn't do the job like drugs did. They stopped everything. They stopped the pain. The eating disorder was probably there before the drugs were, but my choice, if I had to choose one, would be drugs.

But eventually, when I would do drugs to stuff the pain, I'd be high and I'd be crying. I got so miserable that it was a choice between homicide or suicide or my body was just going to die. I just could not live this way. I knew I had to try something else—anything else—just completely change my life.

I knew about this recovery house, so I decided I wanted to go. I guess I knew that I didn't want to be in a hospital, that it wasn't really an option financially and the stay wasn't long enough. The recovery home seemed like the best way to get away and it seemed different from a hospital. It helped me get away from my environment and all my friends. I wanted to start a whole new social group and a whole new life. I stayed there a year.

The first thing was, I just had to admit and accept that I had an eating disorder. For a long time though, I felt like I was being forced—that it wasn't my decision—I abstained, but I still fought it. After I was able to admit and accept it, then I was able to start dealing with it.

I started doing inventories on my history with the disease. Looking at it honestly, for the first time. Looking back with hindsight. When I was going through it, I didn't have a clue. But looking back, I saw the indications and I was able to be honest. I never got to the point where I liked it, though.

With my drug addiction and alcoholism, I'm grateful that I went through it and that I had the experiences and that I was able to get sober, but I was never grateful for being an overeater. I was always embarrassed, and I still am to this day. I hate the fact that this is happening but I just accept it and eat three meals a day. For me—my commitment to recovery—I think I just had to get honest that I had the disease. Drug addiction and alcoholism, at least in my life, were obvious, whereas eating disorders weren't so obvious.

I watched the people around me at the recovery home. I knew that eventually I would move on to something else. I knew I didn't want to settle for the same things most of them were settling for. Hanging around a recovery home after you're out, having menial jobs with no creative fulfillment, having babies and being on welfare—to me that was worse. I'd rather be loaded or dead than have a baby and be on welfare or be a construction worker who lives in a shack and sees the same people every day. I'm sure that some of these people weren't like this, but for me it looked like a nightmare. I just knew that this was not my destiny.

[The year that Laura lived in the recovery home, she passed the California Proficiency Exam, so that she could enter college. She also, became an emancipated minor, meaning as a minor she was legally able to do certain things, such as sign a lease on an apartment.]

At about a year and a half of abstinence, I decided to take acting and singing classes. I was in my first semester of college and decided to drop out and pursue a career in the entertainment industry. I had always wanted to do it but I was always too frightened to step toward it. Once it was validated, I just knew, that somehow, someday, something will happen.

My suggestions to other young people are, first, **just eat three meals and nothing in between.** If you're not doing that, there's really nothing else to start with, no point in doing the rest. Next, get somebody to talk to about it, about the insanity and the stuff going on in your head. Go to O.A. meetings, talk to somebody. Find somebody to talk to that can relate to you. Start writing about it, write out your history.

I just made the commitment to eat three meals a day and nothing in between and to work the 12 Steps and be in recovery. Recovery means being able to free yourself from the compulsion to eat and the obsession with body and weight, and for me, all the other things that go along with eating.

As long as I'm abstinent and sober, I'm facing in the direction of recovery. It doesn't matter where I am, how far down the road of recovery, it's just what direction I'm facing in. I'm trying to do something to recover from all my diseases. I guess the predominant one in my life right now is codependency. Recovery means just trying to do the best I can to work on myself and heading in that direction.

A variety of audio cassette tapes
by Becky L. Jackson are available.
For an order form write or call:

B. L. Jackson
1380 Garnet Avenue, Suite E-336
San Diego, CA 92109

(800) 278-8050

www.dietingrecovery.com